DYING TO LIVE

Embracing Women in the Struggle with HIV/AIDS,
Substance Abuse, and Mental Health Issues

Anjela Thorpe-Moss, Ph.D.

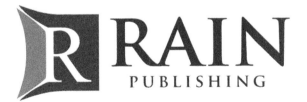

KNIGHTDALE, NORTH CAROLINA

Anjela Thorpe-Moss, Ph.D./Rain Publishing, LLC.
www.RainPublishing.com

Publisher's Note: Names, characters, and places have been changed to protect the identity of some of the subjects in this book.

Dying to Live/ Anjela Thorpe-Moss, Ph.D. -- 1st ed.
ISBN 978-0-9977748-5-6

But I have love.

Looking in the mirror face to face, at the pain that drove me to this place.

Tragedy and shame, Living in agony, Life is not a game.

It's hard facing myself, while running a race with death,

When there's nothing left. Yet I still have love?

How did I get to where the streets are home? I reached outside of purpose now I'm alone.

Existing in a place, an uncomfortable space, drowning in a sea of guilt, living in flesh that hurt has built.

Where I'm running a race with death, Seems like nothing's left, yet I still have love?

Which drug will cause this pain to leave? Which drink will cause my mind to cleave?

To a little time with peace, so I can dream away my life. Alleviate the strife.

I been raped and draped with sin, and lost my way. I've come to the end.

Now I'm running a race with death. Seems like nothing's left.

Yet I still have love?

I find no reason to rejoice, this infirmity was not by choice,

A stronghold has caused my life to turn to bitterness and to discern.

That life entangles with deceit, now I'm in a cage locked up with defeat.

While I'm running a race with death, feeling like there's nothing left.

But I still have love.

No one knows the pain I feel, No one knows the anger I conceal.

Because I went left when I should have went right, down a long tunnel where there was no light.

Someone pull me out of this hole, rescue me and save my soul.

So I can stop running this race with death, and feeling like there's nothing left.

Yet, I still have love.

Then Love spoke and said turn around, and Love set my feet on stable ground.

He was always by my side, took my hand and I began to abide.

In the wonder of his touch, when I felt like falling, Love became my crutch,

And love took away this bitter cup, and told me always to look up.

Rescued me from this race with death, restored the beauty that is myself,

And now I see that I have everything left, I have love.

Written by: Donna Leach Spivey-2015

Dedication

My first dedication of this book is to Rosa M. Ferrell, my biological sister. Rosa prophesied to me in 2000 that God wanted me to write a book, and the title of the book shall be called "Dying to Live." I received that prophecy over 15 years ago; the title has always been hidden in my heart. Over the years I have utilized the title to develop an adolescent pregnancy prevention program titled Dying 2 Live and a curriculum for adolescents called Dying 2 Live to eliminate HIV/AIDS infection among adolescents in our communities.

I would also like to share this dedication with my wonderful husband Wayne D. Moss, Jr. In 2007, God placed Wayne in my life when I could not see my way through. I was in a broken state of mind. Wayne has inspired me to complete my bachelor and master degrees and to further my education in the doctorate program at Walden University as a Health Psychologist. Without his physical, emotional, spiritual, and financial support, I would not have had the courage and opportunity to complete my undergraduate, graduate and Ph.D. programs. My sweet darling husband, I am forever grateful to you.

To my strong and amazing mother, Rose Lee Harris, without God using your birth canal I would not have been here to impact others. Without your Godly teachings in my life, none of this would have been possible. Thank you for your guidance. I have always cared about making you happy and proud of whom I have become. I thank God for allowing my mother Rosa Lee Harris and my biological father John Henry Thorpe (Jake) for birthing a child such as me, a child that is determined to impact and change the lives of God's people with great conviction from God.

To my Step-Father Marshall Ray Harris, thank you for assisting my mother in molding me to become an inspiration to others and for having patience with me, as I grew and took a walk on the path that God had predestined for me. I know that over the years my path brought forth headaches, pain, and sometimes embarrassment, but my walk also brought forth a beautiful son, Travis Oliver Ferrell II, whom I loved at first sight.

Travis, I pray that my legacy lives on in you and Mya Moss. Mya, you are the daughter I always wanted, thanks for giving me an opportunity to pour into you and to empower your life. To my grandsons Cameron Richardson and Joshua Wilkerson, be like your grandmother; be strong, relentless and dedicated to helping others make positive behavior changes.

To my brothers, Henry Thomas Thorpe, James Thorpe, and Tyrone Thorpe, I am proud to be your sister. We are the seeds of Abraham that have blessed Rose Lee Harris. We all are destined for greatness, and I have witnessed God's greatness in each of you.

Brenda Hester, thanks for listening to me throughout the years until the wee hours of the morning.

To one of the most wonderful friends and spiritual sisters I could have ever asked for, Francis Lynn Williams: Lynn, thank you for being my armor bearer. For many years, you supported and assisted me with my vision, and assisted in advocating for those living with HIV/AIDS, substance abuse, and mental health issues. There were many nights that you supported me by staying up late during our grant writing process. Because of our dedication to this cause for so many years our friend base decreased because of the stigma that is attached to HIV/AIDS. Some did not know whether we were infected or not, therefore, they were afraid to be in our presence. We knew we were not infected, but we were fighting for those we loved whom had lost the battle and we were fighting for those we loved so that they would not become infected. To this date, I am still fighting for this cause. To date 0,000,000,000,000 trillion people have been cured of HIV/AIDS.

I am grateful to everyone who invested financially in my doctorate degree program. Your support and dedication allowed me to achieve what God has called me to do. Without that being possible I would not have been comfortable writing this book. Thank you Anita Johnson, Betty Dixon, Blessings Rice, Dr. Brian Fite, Grady Harmon, Henry Thorpe, Mark Anthony Ferrell II, Phyllis Turner, Raheem Olds, Rosa Ferrell, Rose Harris, Susan Gardner, Tempest Hemby, Thurman Daniel, Tracee Goodman, Tyrone Thorpe, and Wayne Moss, Jr.

A special dedication to my spiritual mother Jean A. Taylor (Ma Jean), who preceded us in death in 2007. Ma Jean, thank you for believing in me. You have supported my vision from the first time we met. Not only did you support my vision, but you took me under your wings like one of your own daughters and covered me with your agape love and your prayers. I will never forget you quitting your job to come work in the ministry with me at Glory to Glory House of Refuge. You were the sounding board that kept me, the residents, and my staff balanced. I know you are in heaven watching over each of us.

The Name of the Lord is a Strong Tower: The Righteous Runneth into it, and is safe. Proverbs 18:10. KJV

Why this book was written

Dying to Live was written to empower women living with HIV/AIDS, substance abuse and mental health Issues. Often those that are in the struggle have no one to confide in and do not trust to share their story unless they are led by God and the Holy Spirit to do so. As I wrote, I asked the Holy Spirit to guide me to all truths and help me to reveal things that will free God's people.

As an author and researcher, I humbly wrote this book from my heart's desire to set captives free, to bring healing to God's people, to educate and empower our families, and to eliminate myths that are associated with HIV/AIDS, substance abuse, and mental illness, as well as to eliminate or reduce the increase in HIV/AIDS infections in our communities.

We need to take our communities back; we are responsible for our children and responsible for teaching them how to protect themselves from becoming infected with HIV/AIDS, how to refrain from becoming addicted to substances, and how to manage their lives. These disparities affect many of our African American family members in today's society. We must embrace those in the struggle. We must continue to educate and share stories that prove these are real life issues that are plaguing our African American communities.

The stories in this book are real and the women are currently residing in North Carolina. North Carolina is ranked among the ten states with the highest infection and death rates. As you read these stories I am asking you not to be judgmental. You could have been in the same situation as these women. You may even be in the same situation now and do not know it. There are still men and women who have HIV or AIDS and have not disclosed it to their partners. The only way to know your status is to get tested. Know your status, it is important!

Forward

In an effort to embrace women in the struggle against HIV/AIDS, substance abuse and mental health issues, one would need a strong daily relationship with God. In terms of the church age, we are near the closing of the dispensation of Grace, therefore Christian writers and poets are at an all-time high and they are giving glory to God for their gifts, talents, and what God has done in their lives through the Lord Jesus Christ. I met Angela and her family in the early seventies. Her family became members of Bible Way Church in Raleigh, North Carolina. I worked closely with Angela and her family in nurturing and helping her develop into the young lady she is today. As she matured into a responsible adult, in 1998, she founded and organized a program that provided housing and supportive services to women struggling and living with HIV/AIDS, substance abuse, and mental illness. This became an award winning program and numerous women's lives have been changed because she was a willing vessel for God to use in that season. I am grateful to God that he has allowed Angela the ability to print her personal and innermost thoughts concerning the warfare of disappointment, hurts, tests, trials, tribulations, temptations, persecution, and distress of these women. This book will give them and others that are affected a course of action from chapter to chapter. She will offer solutions to those unexpected challenges that women are faced with day to day.

I present to the reading audiences a new kid on the block, Dr. Angela Thorpe-Moss, whom God has promoted in the Body of Christ for a time such as this. I give honor to God for my friend and spiritual daughter as I congratulate her on her first official literary work, *Dying to Live*.

Betty Woods Dixon, former first lady, childhood mentor
Co-Founder & Establishmentarian
Bibleway Temple, Raleigh, North Carolina

I remember like it was yesterday, Angela called to tell me that God had given her a vision to help women. I don't think initially she knew all that it entailed, but as the days went on her vision became much clearer. In July 1998, The Glory to Glory House of Refuge was birthed and became affectionately known as the Glory House. The Glory House was a home to those who suffered with HIV/AIDS, substance abuse, and mental health issues. This was a home for women from all walks of life and educational backgrounds, but one common dominator the women had was "a second chance." The Glory House was a house of non-judgment. This is where I learned to accept all people where they were and how they are. I saw the community, churches, and families come together to do whatever was needed to ensure that these ladies had all the resources needed to accomplish their goal of obtaining their second chance. I wish I could say that every woman who walked through the doors of the Glory House were transformed. All were not transformed, but all had the same opportunity to make positive behavioral changes. The Glory House is no longer in existence but I love the way Angela has created a way to still reach out to women with her outstanding book, DYING to LIVE. This book will reach women all over the country regardless of race, creed, or color. I feel that everyone will be able to identify with the stories of the ladies that are represented in this book and feel the heart of Angela as she continues to help these women fight for a cure for HIV/AIDS, manage the disease of addiction, and live with their mental illness.

Rosa Thorpe-Ferrell, Sister

For you have risen as the Phoenix rose from the ashes. What was sent to kill you and stop your destiny, only gave you life! The plans of the enemy (Satan) were destroyed. Not only am I proud of you Dr. Angela Moss, so is the Almighty God!

Suzette King, Neighborhood mentor

CONTENTS

CHAPTER ONE

What is HIV/AIDS?

The question, "Where did HIV/AIDS come from?" has always been proposed to me. After teaching basic HIV/AIDS education for many years, the origin of HIV/AIDS has always been a topic of discussion. Most students believed the myth that HIV was created in a laboratory by our government in order to eliminate the African American race. That is a good theory but most individuals do not realize that HIV/AIDS has no barriers. Men, women, and children from all ethnic groups have been infected with this deadly disease. Finding a household in the United States that has not been affected by HIV or AIDS in one way or another is rare. The "West Africa theory" about the origin of HIV/AIDS is that scientists who were hunting chimpanzees in West Africa came in contact with chimpanzees that had a virus called Simian Immunodeficiency Virus (SIV). It was reported that this virus was transmitted to humans when scientists who were hunting them for meat came into contact with infected blood. Many years later, the virus was carried into Africa and then to the United States. In actuality, the onset of HIV was in 1959, when a Kinshasa man in the Congo became infected. However, scientists are not certain how the

Kinshasa man became infected. Blood tests revealed that HIV-1 infection may have come from a single virus in the late 1940's and 50's. Meanwhile, the Government had always known this virus existed in the United States since at least the late 1970's. From 1979 to 1981 doctors on the east and west coast were reporting pneumonia, unusual cancers, and other illnesses by Caucasian male patients who were having sex with other males. This is why early on, HIV was identified as a virus that was spreading among gay white males who were having sex with other males. In 1982 medical providers named this illness that resulted from the virus (AIDS) Acquired Immuno-Deficiency Syndrome. AIDS triggered the government to start tracking newly reported AIDS cases in the United States.

In 1983 scientists were able to discover the virus that caused AIDS. At that time, the virus was called Human T-cell Lymphotropic Virus-type III/Lymphadenopathy-associated virus (HTLV-III/LAV) by international scientists; the name was later changed to HIV. HIV is the virus that can cause AIDS. When an individual has AIDS that means the HIV virus has run its course and it has advanced to the final stages. Individuals at this stage are at risk of contracting other infections that are known to medical providers as opportunistic infections.

Medical treatment and intervention is crucial at this stage. Educating African American Communities about HIV/AIDS is constantly needed. A lot of work has already been done, but there is still a lot more work that needs to be done. In order for our communities to understand how to combat and conquer this pandemic, we must understand the break-down of the virus and the disease.

HIV (Human Immuno-Deficiency Virus) duplicates itself by attaching to cells in the human body. The HIV virus can only be spread from human to human. AIDS is Acquired Immuno-Deficiency Syndrome. AIDS is something that is acquired, that means it has to be given to you. "Immuno" means it affects an individual's immune system. Deficiency means the lack of, and syndrome is a group of symptoms and signs of disease. African-Americans make up 12% of the AIDS infected population in the United States. What is alarming is that African Americans made up more than 46 percent of HIV diagnoses in the year of 2011. Clearly numbers don't lie. African Americans are infected by HIV/AIDS more than any other population in the United States. It is estimated that one in every sixteen African American males and one in every 32 African-American women is at risk of becoming HIV infected in a lifetime. In fact, since the onset of HIV/AIDS in the early 1980's most of the people who died from complications due to AIDS were African Americans. African Americans are the leading population in other types of sexually transmitted disease as well. African-American infection rates versus our counterparts are almost seven times greater for chlamydia, 15 times greater for gonorrhea, and six times greater for contracting syphilis. We also rank the highest in having untreated sexually transmitted diseases particularly those that expose us to a greater risk of obtaining HIV or AIDS. Those are the sexually transmitted diseases that create sores, which puts individuals at a higher risk of becoming infected due to the open sores. In our communities when we think of HIV/AIDS we often think of gay men spreading HIV/AIDS among our communities. 19 percent of the African American men who were HIV infected in 2011, were straight, meaning they were heterosexual men. This could have been your brother, son, father, uncle, husband, boyfriend, cousin or significant other. 89% were women. Research indicated that in

2014, of 1.1 million individuals living with HIV/AIDS, over 506,000 of those individuals are African American. The numbers are not as high as they were in the 80's nonetheless, the numbers are still increasing in African American communities.

I often ask my students and others why the numbers are still increasing in African American communities. They respond by asking if it is contributed to not knowing the transmission modes, or is it contributed to not being able to negotiate condom usage. Knowing how to negotiate condom use and how HIV/AIDS is transmitted are important factors in terms of educating others. Condom negotiation is a learned skillset that empowers partners to encourage condom use and to remain firm in the heat of the moment. The goal is to get their partner to protect themselves as well as you. The outcome is to refrain from having unprotected sex. Individuals have to be clear with their partners about the message of using condoms and protecting themselves. The proper use of condoms can save lives and decrease infection rate in our communities. We must share that HIV/AIDS can be transmitted through blood, semen (cum and pre –cum), rectal secretions, vaginal fluids, and breast milk. In order for someone to become infected via these transmission modes, individuals must have contact with the mucous membrane or damaged tissues. They can also become infected by sharing needles with contaminated blood. Unknowingly, the contaminated blood is injected into an individual's blood stream and can cause HIV which later can convert to AIDS.

The pattern of HIV/AIDS transmission tends to be different among ethnic groups. Both African American males and Caucasian males who engage in same sex behaviors are likely to be infected through sex. Meanwhile, African American men are more likely to share needles than Caucasian men. African

American women are infected more through unprotected heterosexual relationships, on the other hand, Caucasian women are more likely to become infected through sharing needles. Women in general struggle to negotiate condom usage with their partners due to the fear of being accused of having sex with others, and the fear of losing their partners due to trust issues.

Do our communities understand the challenges that have prevented us from decreasing or eliminating this chronic disease? We need to know that these challenges can stem from lack of awareness, poverty, lack of quality affordable healthcare, lack of affordable housing, and lack of prevention education. These barriers play a major role in why African American infection rates are still on the rise and higher than any other ethnic group. HIV/AIDS is the real weapon of destruction in African American communities we are still struggling with fear, stigma, discrimination, phobias, and the undesirable perceptions that plague our people when it comes to getting tested and knowing our status. Those factors put our people at greater risk because we fear rejection from others knowing that we were tested for a potential disease rather than fearing the possibility of becoming infected. Medical providers, outreach workers, social workers, prevention specialists, and those who are human services professionals have become aware of the challenges African American communities have faced, but do community leaders, family matriarchs, and patriarchs know the challenges they face? If family leaders took more time to call our men and women to become accountable in terms of protecting themselves and others from HIV/AIDS, it is my belief that we can impact a lot more people if the disease is always being discussed among our families even in times and settings that seem to be uncomfortable or inappropriate. HIV/AIDS education should always be on our tongue. We must use every opportunity and platform to speak to women, men, adolescents, and not to mention our elderly.

I remember growing up in Raleigh, North Carolina. As teenagers, we learned about sexually transmitted diseases in our high school Health /PE classes. We only knew the world without HIV/AIDS for a short period of time. My son and his generation have not known this world without HIV or AIDS. When he learned about sexually transmitted diseases, HIV and AIDS was the primary topic of discussion taught to his generation.

CHAPTER TWO

Shhh...I Can't Tell Just Anybody He is HIV Positive: A Woman Living in a Mixed Status Relationship

It all began in 1978. I first laid eyes on him in a small church called Bible Way Holiness Church on the corner of Holmes and Bragg streets in the city where I reside. I was only 12 years old at the time; he was a few months older than me. Little did I know, God had already set the path for me, and created a plan for my life. As I became older, I began to become more involved in church activities such as youth leader, youth diocese secretary, and choir member. He was already in the choir. My positions allowed me to spend more time in the church, which led me to being around him and his two brothers a lot more. He and his brothers were always at the church on the weekends, they were very involved in helping in any capacity as their mother was one of the church missionaries. He was the baby of his immediate family which consists of two sisters, two brothers, and himself. I never noticed him as being someone that I wanted in my life. I would get angry when my sister Rosalyn, cousins Jessirae, and Charaline used to tease me about him. I did not like him at the time; he had a huge afro, small face and a skinny nerdy build and wore the same black suit to church every Sunday. He was from the projects, and I was from the suburbs. The projects where he lived seemed like a fun place to live and hang out. It was located two blocks from uptown, and the public bus drove through his neighborhood. They even had an elementary school in their neighborhood. That seemed exciting to me because we did not have access to public transportation in the suburbs, and my mother was not trying to take us anywhere. As much as I wanted to think I was different from him, the facts remained that we were still poor as well. We may not have been as poor as his family was, but we were still poor. The only difference was we had a step-father who was able to put us in our home. As time went on, I was at the age to start noticing boys, and he was at the age to notice girls. After spending more time with his family and hanging in the projects some, I started to develop a huge crush on him, and at the same time I fell in love with Hip Hop. (I always wanted to say that). Hip Hop is the music we used to listen to in the projects such as Eric B. & Rakim, Dougie Fresh, Run DMC, Sugar Hill Gang, Big Daddy Kane, and Kurtis Blow. Trevor was in love with music, rapping, and art, which taught me at the time to have an appreciation for all types of music and the arts. Later he had a profound love for sports, especially football. Fast forward, we were in high school. We were enrolled at different schools and I was simply going through the motion of high school. He was enjoying his high school years as a star athlete. The Caucasian students from his high school viewed him as a superstar from the projects. They used to allow him, his best friend Kurt Kurt, Gary Mo, and Mickey borrow their cars. His school days were exciting since he was a football, track, and basketball star. I always knew that he was going to make it in life. I would sit in the park while he and his friends played basketball at the court for hours. His friends who knew me would tell me that he was going pro and I would be a wealthy woman one day. Whether he became wealthy or not, his destiny was not mine; we were still in our sophomore year of high school. I had my own dreams and ambitions. All we wanted to do at that time was attend football games, sneak into movie theaters, attend parties, sneak a few drinks, and smoke weed. That was the year I was introduced to drugs. I smoked marijuana every weekend. I also had experiences popping pills such as specs and black beauties. I was at the point that I wanted to smoke every time we were together so that we could trip hard off of each other. I thought those were the most exciting days of my adolescent life. He did not realize I was popping pills because I was doing that at school with my Caucasian friends. Late in my high school year, I became pregnant and he was the father of my new child. We both were proud of our new baby, and we were determined to complete our education. I had my baby in April, and I graduated high school in May of that same year. College was not an option for me at that time, and I was afraid. However, he had been awarded a football scholarship to a college in Greensboro, North Carolina. His father drove his mother, him, and me to the orientation at the University. He was excited, I was excited for him, and I was still afraid. I was not going to encourage him to abort his destiny. As we were leaving to come home, he made up some lie to say that the University did not have his scholarship money. Hindsight is always 20/20. At the time that did not seem right, but I did not push the envelope. Later I found out that he did not stay in school because he felt guilty about leaving me back home to raise our child alone. After getting over that hurdle, we began to talk about our next journey, and that was being parents. Two years after high school we decided to get married. I was working a professional job for the county government; he was working in construction and selling drugs. We had our own apartment and we were trying to make it in life by any means necessary. I was afraid of selling drugs, but I would sell bags of marijuana to his friends and mine when he was not there to do so. I was beginning to notice that our relationship was shifting again. He was staying out a lot and partying like it was 1999. That was not acceptable to me. I was a mother and wife. My child was my priority and not him. Although we had been together since the age of 12 years old playing boy and girlfriend, our marriage did not last but two years. We had no other choice but to separate. It was difficult, but we decided that we no longer wanted to live with each other, and we separated. In fact, I came home one day from work and said "I don't want to be married anymore." He replied by saying, "Me too." We immediately ended the marriage. It was difficult but we managed to get through it without hating each other.

Five years passed. I was still working my county government job, and I had purchased my first home, a townhouse. By that time, I had already been a single parent for five years and had accepted the fact that I was a single parent. I continued to work my county government job, and I supplemented my income by working part-time with Namee Barakat, who owned check cashing businesses in the community. I worked as a teller and an assistant manager. I worked various part-time positions within his companies for ten years. Although, I was independent, working, owned my home and had a decent car, I still felt a void in my life. I began dating. I must have had two long-term relationships while I was divorced from my child's father. Those relationships worked for a while, but my heart always told me that at some point we were going to get back together. My latest boyfriend was gunned down in the street by my next-door neighbor and that changed my life. My relationship was over. He was no longer able to stay in the area; his family moved him back to Baltimore because he needed skilled nursing services. After the shooting, I was mentally decompensating for two weeks but the incident eventually caused my life to change in terms of accepting God as my Lord and Savior. By this time, my ex-husband was in a relationship, he had another son, and had progressed in his addiction. He was addicted to marijuana, crack cocaine, and alcohol. I knew that he was not able to assist me in dealing with the emotional turmoil I was in. "Oh but one day." One day my mother came to visit me after the shooting. She was tired of seeing me in the state that I was in. She would come by and say "Huh huh huh, something has to change around here." One day my sister Rosalyn and my mother came over to minister to me. I had been in a daze for two weeks, sitting in the same seat. My baby brother moved in with me for a while to help me take care of my child. Mentally, I was gone. But God! Finally, more than two weeks had passed. My boyfriend at the time had already been transported back to Baltimore; it was time for me to put my life back together again. The problem was I did not know how to do that. My mind was still stuck on the night of the shooting and what I had witnessed. The tape played over and over and over again in my head. It was stuck. That night was imbedded in my head. When my mother came over, she told me that I could no longer sit on that couch and that God was trying to get my attention. She went with me into the bathroom and helped me get a bath. I did all I could to muscle up enough energy to bathe and put on those black and blue polka-dotted flair leg shorts and black tank top. I was finally dressed and ready to attend church. I was finally at church, and the service was good. My mother had been a member of this church for years and I had never known it to have a Caucasian Pentecostal Preacher in the pulpit. He was preaching hard from the depth of his soul, and the audience was praising God like there was no tomorrow. All I can say is if God had returned at that moment we all were going to heaven. Even in all that praise all I wanted was for all the hype to be over with so that I could get in the prayer line. Finally, it was time for the altar call. I walked as far as I could to get to the preacher; I was so weak, I dropped to the floor. I completely crawled the rest of the way to the altar. When I got there on my knees, I asked God how to take away the pain, to help me and to save me, and that night God saved me from myself. Tears were rolling down my face like a stream or river. I could not stop crying. The preacher was praying for everyone individually, and I was thinking, "Can he please get to me?" I was in a state of emergency. It was finally my turn and the preacher whom I had never seen in my life began to minister to me. He was telling me what God expected of me. He asked me to receive God as my Lord and Savior and I accepted God at that very moment. He boldly told me that God said stop praying for a husband; I was already married, and he was going to clean him up, put us back together and we would be in ministry together. By this time, the word on the street was

that my ex-husband was HIV positive, and the girl he was seeing was positive as well. At the time, it was a rumor. Later I
found out that she had a son by him, but the son was not positive. My mind took me back to the rumors about my child's
father, and tears actually started to roll down my face even the
more. I felt like the word from the preacher was not God. I
thought, why would God allow me to get back together with
someone who was HIV positive? These were my exact words
to God, "God you are trying to kill me, why don't you just kill
me right now? I don't want HIV or AIDS." Tears were still
running down my face. I can imagine those who knew me
thought I was crying because God had saved and delivered me.
I was crying because I was scared, and I thought God was trying
to set me up. I cried for the entire service, and when service was
over, I was still crying.

After that enriching service, more time had gone by. I went
about my life working my professional and part-time job as
usual. Days had passed and I thought back on what the preacher
had said to me at the church service. I tried to pass it off as
being nothing but the devil. After a while, it started to surface
in my mind every day. Mind you, the evangelist told me to stop
praying for a husband; God was cleaning up my ex-husband
and putting us back together again. I still did not wish to believe
it. I did not want him to be a part of my life based on his illness
and his drug addiction history. One sunny afternoon, I was on
my way home from work. As I was sitting on the top of the hill
at the stop light before I crossed over a major intersection to get
home, I was staring at the street light and a prison bus went by.
I could have sworn that I saw him on the bus, but he did not see
me. The prison was only a few miles from my house. He must
have been out doing some type of work release job. More

weeks had passed. I was on my way home again sitting at the same stop light that crossed over an intersection to my home. A prison bus slowly passed. I saw him again and we made eye contact with each other. It was an awkward moment for me. I immediately thought God was giving me a sign. After sighting him on the bus two times, I wrote him a letter just to see what had changed in his life and to determine his mindset. At that point, he had been in prison for at least two years, and I had never written him the entire time he was in prison or during any of the times he was locked up before. We began corresponding back and forth and I told him about the goodness of the Lord. I told him about God and how He had changed my life and delivered me from sin and myself. I witnessed to him and convinced him to try my Lord and Savior Jesus Christ. He said, "If God saved you in all your mess I know he can save me." A few weeks later he was released from prison.

In the letters we had talked about getting back together. He asked me if I would take him back, given the circumstances. My heart said no but my mouth said, "I will consider it." I said that so he would not have any false hopes. I am glad I did not allow myself any expectations, because after being released he went back to the projects where he grew up to live with his son's mother. My life went on, and all of a sudden, I started to have very vivid dreams of my ex-husband. God showed me that he was dying, but wanted to live. One night I woke up crying; I had a dream my ex-husband was dead and lying in a casket. He was dressed in a black suit and white shirt. That dream terrified me. The next afternoon, I went to the projects where he and his girlfriend were living. I knocked on the door and she answered. I asked to speak with him, he came out and we talked briefly. I told him of my dreams and asked him about the rumors that he was HIV positive, which he denied. Finally, we had an opportunity to speak one day at his mother's house; she was watching our child. I asked him again about being HIV positive. I told him that he owed me the truth because we have a child together. He then admitted to being positive, and said that he and his son's mother were HIV positive. He stated that he was not sure where he contracted the virus. When he got tested, he was diagnosed with HIV, chlamydia, and syphilis at the same time. He stated he may have contracted it from a one night stand. He said the girl was beautiful, she looked like a supermodel, and they had unprotected sex. His addiction and the mood-altering drugs that were in his system did not allow him to make a rational decision. I invited him to the clinic where I worked.

I opened the doors of the clinic on a Sunday and gave him all the information we had about HIV/AIDS. He stated that he did not know much about the disease, but I was happy to help him and I thanked him for not infecting me. There was a moment where we could have been intimate before I knew he was positive and he refused to be intimate with me. His rejection did not cause me any ill feelings at the time. Later I chalked it up to him and God protecting me. I always knew he was trying to protect me by any means even when we were not together. He was always the kind of person who did not directly want to hurt anyone. If he could protect them, he would.

I was still providing for my child and giving him a life that was joyous and meaningful. One day, my child and I were out rollerblading in my neighborhood and as we looked across the field behind some apartments we saw him. My ex-husband was watching us from afar. My child said mommy, I've seen him before watching us outside. I motioned for him to come closer, and we began to talk. I invited him over for dinner, he stayed for a while, and then he was gone again. We talked almost every day after that day and eventually we began to talk about getting together again. I remember asking him to attend church with me. He said he would, and then a few weeks passed. I remember talking to God just like He was sitting across the room from me. I said, "Lord, the only way I will take my child's father back is if you give me a sign that he has actually changed. Lord, he has to be saved sanctified and filled with your precious Holy Spirit with the evidence of speaking in tongues." Low and behold, he attended church with me. My Pastor was ministering that evening. The praises were high in the church that night. Service was awesome, and people's lives were being changed by the word of the Lord. My pastor had a deliverance ministry. If you walked in one way you would definitely leave feeling free and delivered. My child's father got bold; he walked up to the prayer line. He requested prayer, and God began to prophesy to him through the pastor. My child's father was delivered and set free, but in my mind that did not equate to him having the Holy Ghost. I was excited for him because I knew the power of God. He was beginning to attend every service; when the doors opened to the church he was there. I was already in the habit of going to the church at least five days per week. At some point, I had another talk with the Lord. I said, "Lord, I told you he needed the Holy Ghost and evidence of speaking in tongues." This particular night we had another remarkable deliverance service; my brother was speaking. My child's father was praising God as he had never praised him before. Finally, the spirit of the Lord fell and allowed him to start speaking in tongues. I knew that was a message from God confirming what

I had requested, and He had proven Himself once again to me. My son's father received the Holy Ghost on that night, and the evidence of it by speaking in tongues. That still was not enough for me. I heard the voice of the Lord, and I believed His confirmation, but I needed another sign. "Lord, this man is HIV positive, are you sure you mean that I need to take him back as my husband?"

At that time I still did not answer the voice of the Lord. As months went by my local church was invited to a prophetic church service that was sponsored by Pastor Charles Mellette of Christian Provision Ministries in Sanford, North Carolina. The renowned Prophet Bernard Jordan of Zoe Ministries, New York, NY was presiding. The event was being held at Sanford, North Carolina in the Dennis A. Wicker Convention Center, which has over 17,000 square feet of meeting space. On the night of the event, the Convention Center was packed. Prophet Jordan was ministering, prophesying, and calling people out to say what "thus said the Lord." After a few hours of ministering, Prophet Jordan called out my government name. He told me I needed to come forward; God had a word for me. My stomach began to churn and I was getting what they called bubble guts, that is when you get the feeling of butterflies in your stomach and you are so nervous that you make yourself sick. My then Pastor and all the church members that had accompanied me were looking at me like 'fool, God is talking to you.' I got even the more nervous. I slowly excused myself to the bathroom. On the walk to the bathroom, I said "Lord, I feel like you are talking to me but my name is a common name and there should be at least hundreds of us in this building." I collected myself and returned back to my seat. Another hour passed. The Prophet was still ministering to people when he stopped and called my name again, "Regina." He said my name again, and a lady stood up in the audience. He asked her what her name was, she told him her name was "Gina." He then asked her if her name was short for Regina, she replied by saying no. He said, "God is not talking to you, he is talking to "Regina," and he called my name again, "Regina". I stalled a few more minutes. He said my name again and he also said, "God said that He is not giving up on you, come forward now!" Prophet Jordon put emphasis on NOW. I still refused to answer to the call, so he told the audience how God has used him to spell people's names and call out their social security numbers. The prophet began to spell some of my ex-husband's nickname. At that point I was scared and still not moving. The prophet began to call out the first three numbers of my social security number. I then ran to the altar.

When I got to the altar, I collapsed. Prophet Jordan told his altar workers to stand me up and help me to continue standing, I was weak. He began to minister to me concerning my ex-husband. He spoke so much to me that night. Although I cannot remember all of what God said to me that night, the one thing I have always remembered over the years is that God said He was cleaning my ex-husband up and we were going to be in ministry together. He said our ministry was not going to be the kind of ministry that was popular to the people. Our outreach ministry was going to change lives and set people free. I remember saying, "Thank you, Jesus." I gave Him the highest praise.

I was assisted to my seat as I got myself together. I was still praising God; it was amazing how He could reach me. God knew I was the kind of person that needed show and tell. It was

kind of hard when it came to believing in something or someone that I could not see. I believed and trusted Him but I still
needed proof that He was real in my life and that He honored
my prayers and supplication. From that moment on, I knew that
God loved me and He listened to my hurt, prayers, thoughts,
and concerns. I also learned that I had gained a relationship
with Him because He talked back to me in the most profound
ways.

When I returned home a few days later, I thought about my
encounter with God. I called my ex-husband and told him that
I was willing to take him back regardless of his condition because God told me to. I also told him that God's Word says He
"will heal you of all your diseases." God reminded me of that
scripture in Psalms 103:3 how He forgives all our iniquities and
how He heals all our diseases. That was comfort enough for
me. A week later he was moving into the townhouse that I had
purchased for me and my child. After a few days, I was amazed
by the happiness on my child's face. For my child, it was as if
God had moved into our home. For me I was happy but scared
and nervous. It was always in the back of my mind that during
our separation he had conceived a son and he had a baby
momma. She was never a threat or issue for me. I guess she
knew that dealing with a married man can be unpredictable
even when they have separated or divorced. He would sometimes go and visit his son. I guess most of the women he dealt
with were probably afraid of our connection because we had
known each other since the age of twelve.

Unfortunately, years later he and his son lost her due to complications of AIDS. Although I was not happy that he had
another baby momma, I was remorseful for her death. I thought
that it could have been me, and I thank God that it was not me.

I was told by someone who had been in recovery and struggling with drug addiction for decades that there was a saying in Narcotics Anonymous (NA) that some must die in order for others to live. I am reminded that Jesus died so that we would not die, but have everlasting life. I thought maybe she has finished her course with God and I still have much work to do before he calls me home.

At the time, life seemed on track for me. I was still working my professional job, but I no longer had to work part-time. My child was exceling in school and making friends on our block. As time went by we talked about purchasing a home. The area where I purchased my townhouse was a few blocks from where my ex-husband used to hang out and cop his dope. He would rarely walk down the block to the corner store. Everyone knew him by his nickname. I was still working in the community where there was a high prevalence of homelessness, addiction, prostitution, and other health disparities. God was dealing with me about my ministry. This was in the early 80's when many died on the streets due to complications of AIDS. That is when God gave me the name for the ministry and things were coming together in terms of what my purpose was for that season. The ministry was birthed and called House of Healing. People's lives were being changed. God told me that this was the kind of ministry that would help people live and not die. Psalms 118:17 states, "I shall not die, but live and declare the works of the Lord." I guess this was the birthing of something that I did not know was happening in our life. Just as God had spoken, we were in ministry together and God had cleaned him up and made him a Godly man of valor.

The ministry grew by leaps and bounds. The community embraced the ministry, families were being educated, and people were living longer. There was another shift; God had allowed us to purchase a new home. We were finally moving from the townhouse that was a part of the very community that had claimed his freedom and livelihood for many years. Those same blocks had stolen his continuing education, professional career and most of this fatherhood days. It was a sweet time for him.

We moved into our beautiful three bedroom home with a curved drive way that sat on a hill in a corner lot. The home was immaculate. As you walked in the front door it had a foyer and the master suite was to the right, the living area with fireplace, kitchen, and laundry space was on the other side of the master suite. Upstairs had two additional bedrooms, full-bath and a loft area that overlooked the downstairs living area. The dining areas had French patio doors that led outside to the patio area. We added an invisible screen to the French patio doors and electricity to the hand bricked patio area. My good friend Beverly Townsend's daughter's father Jabo had made the patio area brick by brick.

To me this was how life was supposed to be. This was considered reaping the benefits of the Lord. I was already feeling and looking blessed. After all who wants to follow someone who always looks like they are in the wilderness and never come out? I am reminded of the old school devotional song Ms. Essie Allen use to sing, "Tell me how do you feel when you come out the wilderness yes, come out the wilderness yes." By this time I was working full-time in the ministry and God was providing. I had resigned from my full-time employment and I had to trust God in our ministry. My paycheck was not like receiving a regular paycheck. I worked seventy hours per week for two years and God was making provision for my family. I was just happy that I was given the opportunity to change the lives of others and to empower people to make positive behavior changes. When I left to go home every day, I felt like I had made a difference in someone's life. My clients thought I was helping them; in fact they were helping me to live each day with a man that could have infected me. Over the years, I have learned that HIV/AIDS is no longer a death sentence. Those who desire to live can live. Nowadays, AIDS is considered the same as any other chronic disease. I have not had the fulfillment from my previous employment with a 40 hour week and regular paycheck like I have had working with the women in the program. For the past two years my weeks ended by being blessed and knowing that God will meet my immediate needs. The ministry helped me to deal with living with a man that was HIV positive for over twenty years. I gained strength from the people I served. Someone asked me what was it like living with someone who was HIV positive when I was not positive. Well, the first response was it was scary, and I was terrified for a long time. I often smiled when people saw me because that was my normal demeanor, but inside I was this scared young woman who was wondering if my decision was really God pulling on my heartstrings or was it Satan. I had become obsessive with my body; I was always checking my private parts. I did not want any surprises. I was looking for swollen lymph nodes all over my body, especially under my arms and in the creases of my thigh and under my arm pits. There used to be a time when physicians described the symptoms of HIV/AIDS as having swollen lymph nodes, or having a common cold that would never go away and for most women a yeast infection that felt as if it was from hell. Some of the women I met who were suffering with HIV/AIDS would describe those same symptoms when they were first diagnosed with this disease. Every day was a struggle in my mind. Every day I would look to find something on my body that was not there the day or week before. I allowed the devil to play tricks with my mind for a very long time. Finally, I took authority over my mind. I decreed and declared that I would not become sick with HIV/AIDS; I repeated the words that God promised me back to Him. I often put scriptures in my spirit that spoke to healing but sometimes I still could not get it out of my mind that people were dying, men, women, and children. This was during the critical time that HIV/AIDS seemed like a death sentence to most of the people all over the country. This epidemic had affected and infected many. This was the late 80's or early 90's and people were still dying due to complications of AIDS. Although Trevor did not have AIDS, he was still HIV positive and his condition could have converted to AIDS at any time. I was afraid of becoming infected with HIV or AIDS and that thought haunted me for a long time. I was afraid of having to be alone, or having to bury my longtime friend and husband. I was even more afraid of what people would say about me and my family once they found out his condition. I found myself explaining it to friends and family before they would ask me about his condition and before they could question my health. This whole situation had become daunting to me, I had to constantly pray and remind God of what He said, that He would keep me and heal me of all diseases. Intimacy was no longer the same. In the beginning I was terrified; I was even scared to kiss at times, knowing that kissing was not considered a transmission mode.

As time went on and as I tested hundreds of times, I was convinced that God had kept His word. He was keeping me safe as well as keeping His promise to me. I was confident that I was walking in the promise of God. Who would have made a decision like that knowing it would change their life? Each day, I was reminded of that thorn and each day it allowed me to trust God even more. After a while I almost walked around boasting that I know I am the daughter of the King because He kept me safe and I did not contract the HIV virus. One way to not become infected is to become educated and aware of the transmission modes. We never had unprotected sex. He and I never crossed any boundaries that would cause me to become infected and I never crossed any boundaries that would cause him to contract even a common cold from me that could allow his situation to become detrimental. He was on a number of HIV regimens. At one point they included taking AZT and Crixivan. I could not imagine taking six or more pills per day every eight hours. I watched him do that for years; he wanted to live and not die. Later in his disease progression, he was prescribed other regimens. Those medications slowed down the process of the HIV virus reproducing itself in his system. Later his doctors reported that the HIV virus in his system had become non-detected. I was excited about hearing that report. Did that mean that God healed him? In my mind, I view it as a healing, but I also knew from my professional experience in the healthcare field that it meant that the amount of HIV virus in his blood was lower than the amount that a blood test can measure. That gave me hope and it allowed me to take one step closer to allowing him to become an integral part of our lives.

The biggest challenge for me in terms of living with someone who was HIV positive was always being on point when it came down to protecting myself. The majority of the time, I was conscious of the fact that my husband had contracted the virus. It was important to me that I would not become a statistic under the category of those infected with HIV/AIDS in North Carolina. Over the years, I have learned that people can lead self-directed lives with dignity and hope while living with HIV/AIDS. They must be proactive in getting the rest they need, eat healthier, and refrain from indulging in the use of illicit drugs. In actuality more people are living longer, but the number of HIV/AIDS infections in the Black communities is still rising, numbers don't lie. HIV/AIDS is still classified an epidemic and our Black communities are still losing those who we love. Surprisingly, Black communities seem to think that HIV/AIDS is no longer a major problem due to the media not having it in the forefront as it was a few years ago. The truth of the matter is, we have to remember the numbers are still increasing and our family members have not stopped dying due to complications from AIDS. We have made some strives in educating and informing the Black community about the disease. More and more Black families are embracing their loved ones who are infected with this disease. There was a time when families would not allow infected family members to eat from the same dishes or use the same washer and dryer that they had to use. After being educated about the disease it was easy for me to embrace others, I no longer saw others as being contagious or dangerous to me. I felt free enough to love on them and assure them that they were no different from anyone else. We are all God's children. It was unfortunate that they contracted this awful disease. I cannot imagine how my ex-husband felt about sharing his status with family, friends, and others. In the beginning he was very private about his status.

After God saved him, he began to speak of the goodness of God and how God had kept his body healed and he was able to utilize the activities of his limbs. It took him a long time to be able to openly speak about his disease. After receiving an affirmation and boldness from God, his test had become his testimony and he was happy to profess the goodness of the Lord. He would always bless the Lord for the good reports his doctors were giving him from the infectious disease clinic.

It was a long time before he shared his status with his siblings. I have never heard his sisters or older brother address his issues in my presence. I often wondered if they ever knew anything about their baby brother having the virus. I have never seen or heard of them openly having a discussion about his HIV status. Perhaps it was "out of sight out of mind," I am not sure. Without me in his life at the onset of the disease, he pretty much had to go through the struggle of HIV with limited support, if any. I believe in the beginning, I was his greatest supporter. He is very close to his second older brother; they were able to talk about everything. I am not sure if they had conversations about the virus, but if he talked to any of this siblings his second oldest brother would be the one he would have confided in; they were the best of friends. His older brother has been distant from the family for many years. They would converse when they saw each other, but they did not have a consistent sibling relationship.

People should not allow their loved ones to fight this long battle alone. We need to embrace them in the struggle. We should speak life to their situation. We need to tell them they will not die but live and declare the works of the Lord (Psalms 118:17). It is difficult for most to engage in counseling sessions, therefore, they find themselves without anyone to express their innermost feelings to. Needless to say, I worked full time in the ministry for eleven years. To this day, God has kept his promise to me. I am not HIV positive. If God spoke it, you better believe it. Each time after conducting speaking engagements my closing statement has always been HIV/AIDS DOESN'T ISOLATE PEOPLE, PEOPLE ISOLATE PEOPLE. When you encounter a person who is infected show them love. You cannot imagine their walk in the struggle of HIV/AIDS, substance abuse, or mental health issues. Remember they are "Dying to Live".

Myth- Anyone who is involved with an HIV/AIDS infected individual will become infected.

That is not true; someone who is intimately involved with a person who has HIV/AIDS may not become infected if he or she uses condoms each time and applies them correctly. There is a correct way to apply condoms. If individuals are using latex condoms correctly, it can be 98-99% effective in preventing HIV transmission.

HIV/AIDS Fact- North Carolina is ranked tenth in the nation for the Highest HIV Infection death rate.

Footnote: Smith, M. (2011). Study: N.C. Among 10 States with Highest HIV Infection, Death Rates.

CHAPTER THREE

The Psychological Effects of Dealing with the Loss of a Family Member Due to AIDS Complications

Whenever we have to deal with death, it seems so hard to accept and digest. It has become the most traumatic experience most people would say that they had to deal with during their life-span. God forewarned us that to everything there is a season, and a time to every purpose under the heavens: a time to be born, and a time to die; a time to plant, and a time to pluck up that which is planted (Ecclesiastes 3:1-2). Therefore we can expect to die and expect the death of our loved ones. People have passed away from many health disparities such as cancer, cardio vascular disease, heart attacks, stroke, and diabetes. Why is it so difficult for society to accept the passing of a loved one from AIDS related complications? It is unimaginably difficult for families to deal with the challenges of seeing their loved ones' quality of life diminish due to complications of AIDS, which has caused them to socially isolate.

Social isolation brings on an increased level of stress that will cause individuals to decrease in their overall functioning. What are the psychological effects on an individual who has lost a loved one to AIDS complications? Angel Hunter is a 43 year old African American woman living in Lancaster, Pennsylvania and the mother of my nephew. When she was fifteen she and her family lived in a middle class neighborhood in Garner, North Carolina. I was a high school student at the time. I remember thinking what a prominent middle class family they were. Her father was a fair-skinned, handsome, African American, hardworking family man. Her mother was of a dark smooth chocolate complexion, very well spoken, and always dressed in the finest. Angel and her sister were always finely dressed as well. They had nice things and it appeared they were living a lavish life style. Angel also had an older brother whom I have seen a few times. They all spoke with this elegant northern accent. In my head, I always associated them with the Cosby family. As I grew to know her and her family a little more, they were nothing like I imagined. She describes them as "dysfunctional with the ability to appear functional." The family had moved from Pennsylvania to North Carolina. Her father stayed behind for a while to continue to work and support the family financially. During this time, her mother noticed the funds that were sent home for the family became less and less. Her mother later found out the money was being spent to support his addiction. He was an intravenous heroin addict. Eventually he moved down to join the family. Her mother never had to work, she was a homemaker, and her responsibility was to take care of the children. One morning her father became ill and had to be hospitalized. He stayed in the hospital for a period of time and was diagnosed with AIDS. Angel's mother had to go through a series of testing including for the Human Immunodeficiency Virus (HIV). Her mother found out that she tested positive for HIV. Now her mother suffers from severe depression, alcoholism, and HIV. Angel was too young to fully understand what that meant and how it would impact her family in terms of their livelihood and socio-economic status. As she joyfully came home from school one day, her mother was home. She remembers saying mom, how is dad today? Her mother responded, "They say he has that thing called AIDS." Her mother tried to explain to her as best as she knew how about her father's illness. His disease was progressive and he died two years after he was diagnosed. He never even had an opportunity to leave the hospital. As she wept, she recalled her father wanting to speak to each of them one at a time and in private. He told her that she was the strongest; she had to take care of her new baby and she had to be strong for the family. She held on to those words all these years, even now that she is a mother of three. Angel did not know what those words meant at the time, but as she grew older and as things progressed with her mother, she understood. Angel's mother had no transferable skills, and she never had to be responsible for taking care of the family alone. She was an alcoholic and she battled with depression. After Angel's father passed away, things began to go in a downward spiral for her family. Her mother was drunk and depressed most of the time. I remember Angel having to be home to take on the responsibility of caregiver for her mother and younger sister. She was 15 trying to manage being a teenage mom, a student, a caregiver to her mother, and a parent to her younger sister. She had many roles to fulfill at such a young age. As time went on her mother still continued to heavily drink and she was still battling with depression. She was no longer able to maintain her housing, therefore, she felt it was best to move the family back to Pennsylvania where she had a stronger support system. After moving to Pennsylvania her mother still battled with her addiction and depression off and on, and she was trying to manage her HIV virus. Her mom had times when the virus was non-detected in her system, which means the level of HIV in the blood is below the threshold that detects the amount of virus in the system by a test. This does not constitute that she has been cured.

Good health was still not enough for her mother, she still seemed trapped in her depression. There were times when she was so drunk that she would fall and hurt herself. Angel had gotten tired of the addiction. She had distanced herself from her mother. She stated her mother's "do's made her don'ts better." She was conveying to me that she learned not to do what her mother did with her life. She finds herself being encouraging like her mother would be sometimes. She stated when her mother was sober and stable, she was a good person to talk to, she was empathetic, and she gave good encouraging advice. When she was bad, she was very bad and she would rather not be in her presence when those times occurred.

While reflecting on her mother's story, Angel realized she had more things in common with her mother than she thought. For the first time while preparing to tell her story, she was able to confess, "MY NAME IS ANGEL, and I AM AN ALCO-HOLIC." She has insight and is taking steps to addressing her problems. Now she is dealing with her own alcoholism as well as losing one parent to AIDS complications, and losing another parent to addiction. Losing a parent during childhood can have negative effect on the well-being of the child. One day her mother had a fall after being drunk and she never recovered. Although she had HIV, the virus did not kill her, the conse-quences of her addiction caused her death in March 2016. The death of a parent for any reason is difficult for families, especially when the death includes addiction or AIDS complications. Many families in and outside of the United States have experienced losing parents for these reasons. Nowadays, it is typical for individuals to lose a parent during adulthood rather than childhood which is contributed to individuals having a longer life span. Families still have to deal with the negative perception of the disease and they struggle with the stigma that is associated with HIV and AIDS.

The death of Angel's father to AIDS complications has caused her to internalize a lot of feelings that she has. Research indicates the death of a daughter's father leaves more negative impact on the daughter than the son. In Angel's case she has to be strong for her siblings, children's, nieces, nephews, and grandchildren. They are all she has. She and her family were able to be at her mother's bedside until she took her last breath. Looking back at things she wished she spent more time with her mother instead of feeling so overwhelmed by her addiction. Part of her is happy that her mom has passed on, because now she is in a better place and she does not have to deal with addiction and depression. She is absent from the body but she is now present with the Lord. She finds joy in that alone.

Angel lost both parents and has experienced some significant negative effects. For some, these effects can be an increase in depression, their happiness tends to decrease, they have low self-esteem, they experience a lower level of personal mastery, and overall it lowers their level of psychological well-being. Like Angel's father said, she is strong. She has bounced back from a lot of these factors. Today, she is happy, productive, enjoying her family and grandchildren. She is a psychology student at a local university in Lancaster, PA and she is currently working as an activity coordinator at a local senior nursing facility. Having a loss is always challenging. We should stop viewing death as being final regardless of what they passed away from. When a person passes on to the other side, their death is not final for those who lived in Christ. The word of God says, "Behold, I show you a mystery: We shall not all sleep; but we shall all be changed in a moment, in the twinkling of an eye, at the last trumpet. For the trumpet shall sound, and the dead shall be raised incorruptible, and we shall be changed. For this corruptible must put on incorruption, and this mortal must put on immortality. So when this corruptible shall have put on incorruption, and this mortal shall have put on immortality, then shall be brought to pass the saying that is written: "Death is swallowed up in victory." "O death, where is thy sting? O grave, where is thy victory?" The sting of death is sin, and the strength of sin is the law. But thanks be to God, who giveth us the victory through our Lord Jesus Christ!" I Corinthians 15:51- KJV

HIV/AIDS: Why Is It Not Talked about in our Black Churches? - From a Pastor's Prospective

I believe that God is raising me up in a time such as this to empower churches to make social change that addressees real issues such as HIV/AIDS, substance abuse, and mental health issues across the country with emphasis on communities that have a high prevalence of HIV/AIDS, and bigger populations that struggle with substance abuse and mental health issues. While polling these North Carolina pastors concerning why HIV/AIDS is not regularly addressed among most of the black churches, here is what they had to say.

Bishop William S. Spain,
Glorious Church, Raleigh, North Carolina

HIV/AIDS is somewhat taboo in black churches; we don't like to talk about it. However, it is very necessary to discuss HIV/AIDS in our black churches. Some Pastors are denying that HIV/AIDS is in the church because they are not knowledgeable and they do not have the facts that surround HIV/AIDS education. HIV/AIDS facts have not been heavily taught in many of our black churches. When asked if some Pastors choose not to use the church as a platform to bring awareness to HIV/AIDS, because it may force them to look at their own sexuality, Bishop Spain stated, "That could be one possibility, however, sexuality is not normally talked about in the black churches." He went on to say, "We speak about heaven, we speak of some biblical things; we speak of prosperity, but we don't speak of the things that are hurting us as a people." Pastors are uncomfortable talking about things that are unpopular, or that hurt, but the church talks about things that are popular to their audiences. In other words, the church has become more entertainment than a place to educate, inform, and bring forth healing, deliverance, and display love. In many churches today, anything that is academic or educational is not discussed very much in our pulpits because what is popular for the people is entertainment. We need to touch our communities with the message of love, even the people who are infected with HIV/AIDS that are" Dying to Live".

Bishop Spain has experience dealing with those living with HIV/AIDS in the church after having a narcotics anonymous program for individuals who were struggling with the challenges associated with addiction. As their leader, many of the people in the program respected him and were able to share their status with him. Bishop feels the church has become a place where Pastors have become very selective in terms of what type of people they want in their congregations. The Lord said, "Whosoever will let him come." Sometimes it is difficult to come because the church has so many exclusive clubs. The ultimate message should be love and how it covers a multitude of sins.

"Charity suffereth long, and is kind; charity envieth not; charity vaunteth not itself, is not puffed up". I Corinthians 13:4(KJV)

Bishop James E. Thorpe,
Former Pastor of Rehoboth Family Worship Center,
Raleigh, North Carolina

When Bishop Thorpe was asked why HIV/AIDS is not talked about regularly in black churches, he kindly responded by stating that fear is a major factor for not speaking out concerning HIV/AIDS in some black churches. He also stated that you never know what a Pastor does behind closed doors, and if he or she is living a double life then they might be afraid of the possibility of having the disease themselves and dealing the stigma associated with it. Another issue is that some churches have become very guarded about discussing topics of sexuality, and the consequences that reckless sexual behavior breeds. He instilled in his children at an early age that if you are not going to wait until you are married to engage in sex, which is almost unheard of in today's society and his culture, then you need to practice protecting yourself by using safer sex methods. Reestablishing the respect for our bodies is a major issue that can be addressed. He has always told his sons and daughters that once you give someone your body, you have given them everything. Some of the modern day churches don't teach abstinence like it was taught when Bishop Thorpe was coming up in the church. The church has to refocus on getting back to the plan of God, cry loud and spare not, but do it in love and the hearers will better adhere to the warning cry. Another issue is the church fails miserably at treating the whole individual. Ministries are supposed to be holistic, treating the mind, body, and the soul of man. When Pastors don't have a holistic approach in terms of ministry, there will always be an imbalance among the lives of individuals they serve in our congregations. We don't talk about the mechanics of the body, and although you are saved woman and men, some still have urges and desires that have not been addressed. They are left perplexed and confused about what to do, and are still making the wrong decisions due to lack of information and being misinformed. When Bishop Thorpe looks at the state of the church and the people who are dying spiritually, it is really upsetting to him. He has often asked himself, why are the numbers still increasing and why are people still struggling with these issues, as a church? Are we doing a good job dealing with the holistic person? Are we really treating the whole man? Are individuals getting all they need in one service or church? At best the church should help you to see that you need help whether it is in the mind, body, or the soul. In reality, most churches would be blessed to have a person from their congregation on staff that has the skill-set to serve the mentally ill in their congregations, and stop passing them off as demons. Wake up churches, wake up Pastors, HIV/AIDS, substance abuse, and mental illness are diseases and they need to be regularly addressed in our churches and communities.

"Now may the God of peace make you holy in every way, and may your whole spirit and soul and body be kept blameless until our Lord Jesus Christ comes again. God will make this happen, for he who calls you is faithful."

1 Thessalonians 5:23-24 (NIV)

Bishop Michael Ferrell,
Breakout Ministries, Charlotte, North Carolina

One of the reasons that it is difficult for Pastors to use the church platform for HIV/AIDS awareness in some black churches is because of ignorance, and they have not been educated about the disease and the various myths that people have established in the minds of the individuals. Some are still afraid of the mode of transmission; they still seem to think they can get it by sitting near someone, or shaking their hand or giving a Godly hug. Another perspective is because most black churches have not engaged in the preventive work regarding HIV/AIDS. Therefore, many Pastors may be discouraged because they feel they are not well prepared enough to discuss that issue among the church. Many Pastors tried to sensationalize or spiritualize that topic when talking about HIV/AIDS by saying the Lord is going to do certain things. What is the action plan? What we can do to help those who come through our church doors that are broken and are struggling with HIV/AIDS, how we should embrace them instead of running them off? That is the question most pastors should be asking themselves. Some seem to think because the government and our legislation have endorsed same-sex marriages that HIV/AIDS is the retribution of one's sexual behavior, and the lifestyle has become more open and pervasive. The gates have been open; now we have to figure out how to help those who are affected and infected with HIV/AIDS. This is someone's child. Bishop Ferrell was reminded of those people in the Bible who had leprosy. The people were putting individuals in certain communities, and supplying them with food and resources, but they could not come into their communities. Jesus wanted to break that because that was not His intention. That was man's solution and not God's plan because man did not have a valid solution to help the people who were infected with leprosy. The black churches are so behind. They are trying to figure out how to help people that are already in the church and then Pastors bring on the dynamics of HIV/AIDS and other health disparities that can be even the more challenging for a pastor to take on. The black churches are misinformed because they are trying to deal with modalities like making sure the rent is going to get paid or is the pastor going to get paid? Bishop Ferrell believes that the pastors should direct individuals to the right resources if they are not equipped to deal with issues such as HIV/AIDS and other health disparities in the church. Some pastors want to help, but they want to help certain types of people. Those who are suffering from HIV/AIDS, substance abuse, and mental health issues are not in the vision of the ministry. Therefore, they do not have a desire to address those problems. This is why the black churches are suffering when it comes to helping those living with HIV/AIDS. These churches are not educated about the topic, they have a low tolerance, and they are not willing to be objective and learn what needs to be done in their community. Bishop Ferrell believes that pastors must be open to bringing a holistic message that helps everybody, not somebody. Pastors need to be equipped, since after dealing with HIV/AIDS, there are going to be other chronic issues the church is going to deal with. As pastors, it is important to become educated and surround yourself with others who are well informed. Bishop Ferrell has a firm conviction that with the wisdom of God, we will be able to incorporate helping communities live again.

Apostle Annie S. Hinnant
Power of Praise Tabernacle of Deliverance
Benson, North Carolina.

One reason some Pastors in black churches are not talking about HIV/AIDS regularly is because they have not been affected by HIV/AIDS. For example, if someone has not experienced dealing with the death of a loved one, they do not know what that experience is like. When you are standing on the outside looking inside of a situation, it is very hard to put your whole heart into it because the situation doesn't impact you directly. Apostle Hinnant concurred that HIV/AIDS is definitely an issue that needs to be regularly addressed in black churches and she is first to repent because she is not affected by this issue in her congregation as far as she knows. She has not used the church platform to address this issue, but she does address other health disparities among her congregation. However, her church is known for their healing and deliverance power. The church once had a visitor who reported he was healed from AIDS as a result of the prayers that went forward at Power of Praise Tabernacle of Deliverance. Apostle Hinnant wants everyone to know that these are serious issues, people are still dying, and this issue needs to be addressed across our pulpits regularly.

Apostle/Senior Pastor Monica Lee
The Ark of the Covenant Church
Cary, North Carolina

Pastor Lee believes that HIV/AIDS is not being addressed regularly based on a lot of factors, including perception. She feels that most congregations still have a false perception about the transmission modes and how HIV/AIDS is attached to sexually transmitted diseases. She stated there is a high number of persons in the church is infected and affected by HIV/AIDS. They are not comfortable about openly exposing themselves due to the fear of being ostracized and isolated from those they love. She went on to say that the church is not ready to deal with controversial topics such as sex in the church, so the church tried to stick to the core value of belief according to the bible. Most churches are not knowledgeable or equipped to deal with health disparities in the church including saints who struggle with substance abuse and mental health issues. Some pastors do not deal with those issues because it does not personally impact them directly or they do not want to deal with the stigma that is attached to HIV/AIDS, substance abuse, and mental health issues. Pastor Lee wants to encourage pastors to address the issues in the church. Let's talk about those issues, it is essential to having a healthier lifestyle.

Prophetess Jacki London
Pillar of Fire Worship Center
Warsaw, North Carolina

When Prophetess London was asked what God saying is to the church about people who are dealing with HIV/AIDS, substance abuse and mental health issues, she shared that God is saying to tell His people to humble themselves and pray and seek His face; He will heal the land. We should not be concerned with what people have and cause them to lose sight of God, we should be concerned about what God can do in order to bring healing and restoration to them. She believes the church has forgotten to love and has lost its first love. The church needs to get back to seeing people through the eyes of God. Regardless of their alternative life styles, we still need to see people as souls. These health disparities are real outside and inside the church and they must be addressed so the people of God can be healed. Prayer changes everything, God can heal all types of illness. Illnesses are not a curse from God. God is consistent in his theology. He is a healer! God loves those who are struggling with HIV/AIDS, substance abuse, and mental health issues, so should the people of God.

Pastor Melita Thorpe
Greater Power and Praise Ministry
Durham, North Carolina

Pastor Thorpe informed me that in her personal opinion, the black churches have gotten away from deliverance in general. They have gotten away from the real issues that affect the body of Christ. She believes that HIV/AIDS is not readily talked about among black pastors in the church because pastors do not want their colleagues to look at them in a different light. As pastors, most of the time when they address an issue, it means that issue is in their congregation or that is the population they are targeting. If pastors don't target the sick then what purpose do they have? Therefore, they are not serving the community like they should. When Jesus was on earth in the flesh, He was not in the churches, he was out in the community teaching and doing the work of His father. Multitudes of people were following Jesus. He was not concerned about what the people said or what they thought of him, He was among all people. The only thing He was concerned about was the Father Who sent Him. Many pastors have gotten away from the work that our Father has sent us to do. Pastors have become more worried about how they are viewed and what people think of them, rather than being concerned about the souls of people. When you become concerned about people's souls that means that you are concerned about their wellbeing. You want to know what got them to the state they are in. For some pastors that takes work, and most pastors do not want to do the work of going out into communities, compelling people, and showing them a better way of life. In doing so, Pastors have to be open, honest, and not ashamed of where God has brought them from because it could have been them living with HIV/AIDS, substance abuse, and mental health issues, "But God." Until pastors are not afraid or ashamed of where they came from, they will not be able to help others, to prevent them from falling into the same pit. Some things are preventable and pastors have to be open to sharing our stories to prevent and compel others. Pastors have to put in the work to prevent some things from happening to others. Pastor Thorpe's message to pastors who are not addressing real issues that are attacking our people is they need to get back to doing what God has called them to do. God did not call them to a popularity contest; he did not call them to gain members, he called them to the multitudes to compel men and women to come to Christ. Pastor Thorpe says she is excited about doing her part in the body of Christ, but if she does not compel her brothers, sisters, and colleagues to do their parts, that means that she has not truly done her part.

And the lord said unto the servant, Go out into the highways and hedges, and compel them to come in, that my house may be filled. Matthew 22:23 (KJV)

The LORD hath appeared of old unto me, saying, Yea, I have loved thee with an everlasting love: therefore with loving-kindness have I drawn thee. Jeremiah 31:3(KVJ)

Pastor Kenneth Hester
New Life Community Church,
Oxford, North Carolina

Pastor Hester indicated that one major reason HIV/AIDS is not being discussed in our black churches is because of the lack of education on the topic. He stated when talking about HIV/AIDS, one has to be equipped with the knowledge of addressing the topic, because the people of God are going to ask questions. Pastors need to be confident with the answers they are giving, and they need to be conveying the right message. If pastors are not educated on the topic of HIV/AIDS, they should consider not discussing it until they become educated and learn the facts. Another issue that may be a barrier is that pastors who are in communities with a low occurrence of HIV/AIDS cases may not be as forthcoming about discussing the topic because the issue never comes up in the church, and he or she feels the church is not being impacted by the disease. However, Pastor Hester does believe that HIV/AIDS needs to be addressed regularly in churches all over the country and the community, especially those communities that have a high prevalence rate of HIV/AIDS. He believes that these topics will have a greater impact if they are addressed at youth conferences and other events that are held where the community has come together to fellowship. Pastor Hester shared that he asked himself, how many pastors even know what the acronym HIV/AIDS means? Pastor Hester said he can guarantee that 8 out of 10 Pastors do not know what those acronyms stand for. He humbly reminded me of the scripture in Matthew 15:30, "and great multitudes came unto him, having with them those that were lame, blind, dumb, maimed, and many others, and cast them down at Jesus' feet; and he healed them." Someone in that group probably had an illness similar to AIDS. He believes that many people are not being healed of HIV/AIDS and other health disparities to include substance abuse and mental health issues due to their faith. If they can believe it, God can truly heal them. Healing comes with faith. God healed the woman in the bible who had an issue of blood for many years because of her faith. She believed that God could heal her. It was her faith that moved God. Pastor Hester would like to encourage pastors who are not addressing these issues to let the people know that God can do all things; He is bigger than any situation that attacks their life. Pastors need to bring someone into our churches who is equipped and educated to talk about HIV/AIDS and other health disparities.

"And Jesus departed from thence, and came nigh unto the Sea of Galilee; and went up into a mountain, and sat down there. And great multitudes came unto him, having with them those that were lame, blind, dumb, maimed, and many others, and cast them down at Jesus' feet; and he healed them". Matthew 15:29 (KJV)

Pastor Robert Mason
Greater Love Worship Center
Durham, North Carolina

Pastor Mason's main belief is that pastors in the body of Christ do not touch on HIV/AIDS in African American churches because it is a faith issue. Many people have been affected and infected by this pandemic that has claimed the lives of many. Some pastors and churches do not address this topic due to operating in fear. If God healed leprosy in the Bible surely he can heal HIV and AIDS. They should be able to proclaim faith so that others can be healed. Some pastors have moved from preaching faith and the resurrection power of Jesus Christ to preaching clichés. When pastors start preaching clichés, they start plagiarizing other people's sermons which causes them to move away from the core value of the bible. AIDS is similar to cancer in terms of how the disease attacks the human body. This pandemic has impacted many countries including the Unites States. Pastor Mason would like to encourage others "not to tell God how big their problems are, but tell your problems how big your GOD is."

Most of the pastors feel that these issues are a reality and that the church needs to become educated and equipped to handle them. They need to be taught on the preventive measures people can take to protect themselves from substance abuse, HIV/AIDS, and other health disparities. These pastors also believe the church needs to have conversations about addiction, sex, and the stigma that is attached to sexually transmitted diseases. These were the issues that distinctly stuck out among the Pastors in North Carolina that were polled. They all agreed that church should serve as platform to reconcile others to Christ, to address health disparities, and to encourage prevention, education, and to promote wholeness in the body of Christ.

CHAPTER FIVE

He Loved me Regardless of my Illness

Meet Tisa, she is a 50 year old African American woman. She grew up in a small town in Inkster, Michigan which is not that far from Detroit. She is the oldest of three children, and the only girl. Tisa's mom gave birth to her at the age of sixteen. When she was born it was against all family rules and totally against what the family stood for to be a pregnant teenager. After Tisa's grandparents found out her mother was pregnant, her grandparents put her mother out of the home and demanded that the baby stay with them. Tisa's grandparents raised her from a baby until she was promoted to the sixth grade. Tisa described those days as living a "pretty normal life". She said her grandmother always purchased anything she wanted. Her grandmother even purchased things for her that she did not ask for. Tisa remembered her life as being somewhat sheltered, her grandmother did not allow her to do too much. Tisa has always known who her mother was, they were always close, but she never lived with her until she was in the sixth grade. Even now people think she and her mother are sisters because they look so much alike. Tisa's mother and biological father had been married for many years before they were divorced when Tisa was nine years of age. Tisa was happy to learn of their divorce before moving in with her mother. Her mom was in an extremely abusive marriage, and as a small child she witnessed many of her mother's beatings. In her mind as a child she had this grandiose attitude and would think to herself, maybe her mother will leave when she is tired of the beatings. She believed that her mother's abusive relationship was why she had to be raised by her grandparents for so long. They did not want her to be in an environment with so much physical and emotional abuse. In high school, she was a "B" average student with a very small friend base. Her high school years were fun times for her; she was involved in sports. She had been telling her mother and other family members that after high school she was leaving, but it appeared that no one believed her. She kept repeating it for many months. Her mother said that if she decided to join the military, she would not sign the papers, so Tisa enrolled in the delayed entry program. The plan was to graduate in June, 1984, turn eighteen in August, 1984 and leave for the military in May, 1985, and that is what she did. She reminded her mother that she did not need her signature; she would be of appropriate age in a few months. Her mom was saddened and disappointed about her decision to join the military, in fact, she never believed that she was leaving the state. After graduating from high school in 1984, she joined the military in May, 1985. She kept telling herself she had to go; she had been in the State of Michigan for eighteen years and she just could not stay around there any longer, so off to the military she went. She saw no future in staying in Inkster, Michigan. There were no jobs, no opportunity for college, and she was determined that she was not going to hang around and do nothing, among other things that led her to flee her home state and city. There was urgency in her spirit that was telling her that she had to go. She did her basic training in Fort Dixon, New Jersey, her schooling in Fort Belvoir, Maryland, and she was stationed in Fort Bragg, North Carolina. She was thinking, "Oh my God North Carolina; I really did not want to be stationed in North Carolina of all the places on this planet." Fort Bragg was the last place she wanted to be and the only place she ended up being stationed. She spent eight long unwanted years in Fort Bragg.

In the military, they had started a procedure to begin HIV/AIDS testing for the soldiers, which is how Tisa learned of her HIV positive status. She was nineteen years of age. She thinks she contracted the virus from someone who did not know they were infected or just did not care to tell her they were infected. After getting over the shock and crying for two months, Tisa had a conversation with God. She said, "Ok God it is just me and you, let's ride, I have too much that I need to do." She was very athletic and played softball, volleyball, and flag football in the military. During her high school years, she played basketball, volleyball, and track. While in the military, she met the man of her dreams; he was in the process of exiting the military. She was glad because he was in infantry and they stay gone too long.

They met at a night club shortly after he had returned home from Iraq. While in the club he kept staring at her, which gave her a very uncomfortable feeling because she hates to be stared at. She had to find out what he was staring at so she walked to him from across the room. She asked him if something was out of place or was something wrong. Her grandmother always told her, "If you're going to be staring at someone, you might as well speak." He told her that he really wanted her. She kept telling him that he really did not want her. He insisted. She told him if he wanted her he had to know everything about her and what he was getting into. She then said, "This is what you need to know. I am HIV positive." He sat in silence for a minute. After he collected himself, his response was, "Well everyone has to die of something." She stressed to him, "You did hear what I said?" He responded again by saying "Yes, I heard what you said." She responded, "Alright as long as you know what you are getting into."

The two married in 1995 and have now been married twenty years and together twenty-four years. Her husband stopped using condoms after they got married, which was a shock to her. She did not like his decision, but he would shush her and say, "We're married now." She was aware of the risk, and had been educated on the different strands of the virus and how important negotiation of condom use is even when your partner is positive. Tisa knew the consequences of two HIV positive individuals having unprotected sex. She knew there are different strains of the HIV virus and an individual who has unprotected sex and is positive can become infected with another strain of the virus. Superinfection can occur but medical providers are not certain of the frequency of this happening. Individuals can possibly become more ill after obtaining a second strain of the virus. She was upset for a little while in terms of possibly making her husband sick, but she had gotten to the point of comforting herself by saying this is what he wanted to do. She thought that if he was not fearful about contracting the virus, why should she be? God did not give her the spirit of fear, but of love, power, and a sound mind. Two years after being married, her new husband contracted the virus.

Tisa also wanted a baby, and she knew by being HIV positive her baby could potentially become infected. Her medical providers had described the risk to her and the probability of her unborn child becoming infected. After looking back, hindsight is always 20/20. Tisa believes that she was very selfish to bring a child into this world knowing there is a high chance her unborn child could be born HIV positive, but she took that risk and in 1993, she gave birth to a beautiful baby boy. Her son was one of the children in North Carolina who was born with HIV and will be on medication for his lifespan. He is currently 22 years old and in good health. Today, when he gets sick and struggles with being HIV positive she constantly blames herself for birthing a child knowing that he would probably be HIV positive.

Tisa's husband never talks about being HIV positive nor does he talk about his son being HIV positive. It is like there is a pink elephant in the room. The topic is never up for discussion. They are living with it but they never talk about it among themselves. Her husband and son are very private people. Tisa loves telling her story, but she cannot openly tell her story without exposing her son and his father and neither are in agreement with her doing that.

After reflecting on the day Tisa heard the words, "You are HIV positive," she remembers being fearful and asking, "Are you serious?" She had no indication that something detrimental was wrong with her, no signs, symptoms, or warnings, she was in perfect health. The next thought for her was, "Oh Lord, how am I going to tell my mother?" Tisa asked the medical providers to share her status with her mother because she was in no emotional shape to do it. When the medical provider informed Tisa's mother that she was HIV positive she just kept encouraging her daughter that everything was going to be alright and she could do this. She could live with this virus and embrace the struggles of living with HIV/AIDS.

In the beginning, the hardest part of knowing she was HIV positive was wondering if she was going to be alone without a companion, a husband, or significant other for the rest of her life. The thought of dying was not a fearful issue for her, she had seen people live with HIV/AIDS for many years. Although she had been in church for many years and was raised in the church, no one really knew of her status beside her mother and very few other people. After her grandfather died she rededicated herself back to God and started going to church again consistently. She told her pastor of her condition. This was later after the onset of HIV/AIDS when people, especially African Americans were afraid of HIV/AIDS and the stigma was so obvious. Fortunately, her pastor did not treat her any differently than the other church members. Today a few of her close friends know her status and a few people at her church know her status but she believes that they do not remember that she shared that with them. When she disclosed her status to church folks two to three years ago, they embraced her in the struggle of HIV/AIDS. Some stated they did not know and that they could not look at her and tell that she was HIV positive; some did not believe her story and thought that she was lying. She had to convince them she was not lying. She was happy to hear their concerns and comments. She plans to live a very long time with HIV/AIDS. She believes had she shared her story with people in the early 1980's their behavior would have been different from today. They would probably have given her strange looks, would have withdrawn from her touch, and refrained from hugging or kissing her. Tisa feels that when people do not want to deal with her after knowing her status, it is their problem, not hers and they need to be educated concerning HIV and AIDS. She lives a normal life with HIV; she takes her medication at night, and she goes to work every day.

There are some bad days. She deals with episodes of depression. When those depression episodes hit she does not want to be bothered with people. She feels her depression came after the onset of HIV/AIDS in her life. There are moments when she thinks it is pointless to deal with the struggle of HIV/AIDS; she's had crying spells when others are not around. She does not struggle much with HIV but when she does have those moments, usually no one sees it.

Her biggest personal challenges dealing with HIV to date were informing her mom and dealing with her son having frequent visits in and out of the hospital. He has been struggling with the virus. He is only 22 years old and is constantly in and out of the hospital. He takes eight different HIV regimens per day. She personally holds herself responsible for his condition and is fearful of losing him. She frequently asks herself, what has she done and why did she make a decision to bring a child into the world knowing the child would probably contract HIV? She knew the risk but she wanted a baby so badly. She had counted up the cost but now she has to live with the consequences of assisting her son as he struggles with the virus every day of his life. During the time she was pregnant, the doctors were not giving mothers Zidovudine, Retroviro (AZT) or providing AZT to the child for months after being born. Zidovudine, Retrovior (AZT) is an anti-HIV drug that is supposed to

slow down or prevent damage to the immune system, and reduce the risk of developing AIDS-related illnesses.

Today, Tisa says she has learned that God does things that
we do not understand. As long as she has good health and God
wakes her up every morning she is good. She is just glad that
God has allowed her, her husband and her son just one more
day. What surprised her about HIV/AIDS is that people can live
long, healthy lives with dignity and hope. Since being tested
positive for HIV her perspective has changed, she has become
more understanding, and she is constantly educating herself in
terms of HIV/AIDS and other opportunistic infections. Tisa's
church does a health month, so she wanted to tell her story, but
one of the church mothers gave her advice not to share her story
because some people will not understand and embrace her testimony. This is unfortunate because our real testimonies can
impact lives, heal others, and set captives free.

Many churches today cannot handle our real testimonies;
they are afraid of dealing with real issues. They are fine as long
as the pastors are teaching and prophesying prosperity, houses
and cars. Most people in churches are afraid of people with ter-
minal illness, mental health, and substance abuse issues. Being
different or having a different personal struggle that others are
not used to being around can sometimes cause isolation for the
individual. When it comes to mental illness and substance
abuse among the saints, stigmas are still associated with these
types of health disparities. Even years later since the onset of
HIV/AIDS there is still a strong stigma that is attached to
HIV/AIDS. Some people are still afraid of this disease. They
do not believe that the current identifiable transmission modes
are the only ways of contracting HIV/AIDS. Some think that

the government has purposely not disclosed other ways of contracting HIV/AIDS. When Tisa was first diagnosed in early 1985, she lost a lot of friends. She heard rumors of the things people were saying about her. People need to know the truth about HIV/AIDS so they can gain understanding before dealing with those infected and affected by HIV/AIDS. They must know the difference between HIV and AIDS and learn the infection modes, which is ways people can become infected. Tisa believes that psychotherapy counseling concerning HIV/AIDS is good for some but she depends on the church for her healing.

Due to living a very sheltered life she became promiscuous when she was younger and engaged in unprotected sex. To her HIV was the consequence of her sin, however, God did not give her HIV. Her promiscuous behavior led her to having unprotected sex, which led to her becoming HIV positive. Being in a broken family may have bearing on how Tisa's life turned out, but she is not sure about that. She never knew her father, although the man who was on her birth certificate attended the same church as she. One day, she told him that he was on her birth certificate; he said her mother was lying and he was not her biological father. She later tried to get the truth out of his sister, but she never confirmed or denied that her brother was Tisa's father. That moment left her crushed. Later he passed away and she never got to know the truth or was able to have a relationship with her father. Today, Tisa holds a bachelor's degree in psychology. She is a dedicated disciple of Christ, a loving mother and wife, she is learning sign language as a second language, furthering her education, and she is a faithful usher at her local church.

Myth- A person can get infected from mosquitoes after they have bitten an HIV/AIDS infected person.

That is not true; Studies have shown that there is no evidence that supports this myth. HIV cannot live a long time inside the body of an insect. When insects bite an individual they do not inject the blood of the person that they have recently bitten.

HIV/AIDS Facts - Nearly half of the people living with HIV in the U.S. reside in the South.

Footnote: Smith, M. (2011). Study: N.C. Among 10 States with Highest HIV Infection, Death Rates.

CHAPTER SIX

Substance Abuse and Addiction

As I was reflecting back on the times when I was a young child, I remembered when my maternal grandmother hosted house parties where her friends and family members would come over. They would be drinking, listening to music, frying chicken, and playing cards. It seems as if they were having the best time of their lives fellowshipping with each other. I was always somewhere nearby, lingering in the background listening to the adults and occasionally stealing a few beers from under the card table. It's funny, to this day I do not like alcoholic beverages, and it is very rare that I will take a drink. Alcohol was never appealing to me as an adult. I remember seeing people getting drunk, passing out but I never remembered anyone using substances outside of alcohol. Researchers have traced the history of drug abuse and addiction back as early as the 1970's and 1980's. In the early 1980's people started to discover a new substance on the East and West Coast. That was around the time I was experimenting with using marijuana and dropping a few black beauties (pill containing amphetamines and dextroamphetamines). I had heard about crack cocaine but I was always afraid to try it, especially after hearing about the famous basketball star Len Bias dying after using cocaine in 1986. That was the end of my substance abuse season; I chose to live and not die. Dr. Edward Feldmann who was a neurologist at Brown University in Rhode Island spoke about how the cocaine probably killed Len by causing his brain and heart to be stressed. That was enough for me but it was not enough to cause others to not fall under the spell of addiction. The government is aware of the drug problems in the United States and they have put stricter laws in place. They say they are fighting the War on Drugs, while many people are still battling with addiction. Drugs are still prevalent on our streets, and they are easily accessible if one is seeking to find them. The following women have allowed me to tell their stories. They are troopers when it comes to making positive life style changes to regain their lives. Try to be in a no judgment zone by thinking about how this could have been you or someone you love. These stories may even be about someone you love. These women are assisting me in uncovering these health disparities to open the eyes of others, to educate and to bring awareness of these topics to our churches, organizations, and communities.

CHAPTER SEVEN

Substance Abuse Changed my Life, a Woman in Long-term Recovery

Allow me to introduce Frances Lynn Williams. She is a woman in long-term recovery. After working as my assistant for many years, Lynn became my best friend. Lynn was born May 6, 1957, to a military family in Fort Jackson South Carolina. Her father was 47 years old when she was born and he always gave her everything she wanted. She was his only child, and he spoiled her. Her mother had another child by a previous marriage. He is Lynn's brother, and he is fifteen years older than her. She and her brother never grew up in the same house. When her mom married her dad her brother chose to stay in Hampton, Virginia with their grandmother. Lynn's family moved around a lot. They were in Georgia, Texas, and Germany. She and her elder brother did not live in the same city until she was ten years of age. Her father retired as a chef from the military after serving 27 years with 100 percent disability and her mom was a stay-at-home mom until her father retired. After her father retired, Lynn's mom went to work at Langley

Air Force base in the dining hall doing various duties. When her parents moved to Hampton, Virginia, they stayed with her maternal grandmother for three to four months while their home was being built. Her parents purchased a brand new home which was quite an accomplishment for Lynn's family in 1967. Their net family income was $3,000.00 per month, a lot of money in those days. Lynn received a check which was a portion of her father's disability income as long as she was in school. Lynn and her family finally moved into their home located in a historic Aberdeen subdivision. This was the first time Lynn had experienced going to a predominately black school, and it was the first time she felt like she was different. Lynn had always gone to military schools on military bases. When she first started school she lived in Germany. The school was located on the military base, and she was the only Black American child in the class at that time. After moving to Hampton Virginia, to live with her grandmother until their home was built, she still attended a predominately white school. When she got to Aberdeen Elementary school, this is when she first experienced emotional abuse, particularly from her peers. According to the National Historic Places listing in Hampton, Virginia, Aberdeen was a historic landmark in Hampton Virginia. It was the only community in Hampton, Virginia where the land was owned, built, and nurtured by Black Americans. Today it is a historic landmark in Hampton, Virginia. Although the neighborhood was welcoming, the school was very frightening. The students saw her coming in new and becoming the teacher's pet. This stemmed from her raising her hand and knowing all the answers to the teacher's questions. The other students decided not to like her. In her previous school, the students raced to raise their hands because quite a few student knew the answers. At Aberdeen Elementary, it was not like that. The teachers saw her as smart, and expected her to know the answers, but knowing the answers was not favorable among her peers at Aberdeen Elementary. Lynn knew all the answers because she had learned those lessons at her previous school. The first week of attending Aberdeen Elementary school she hated it. She cried, she was called out of her name by her peers, and they hated her because she was smart, skinny, and light skinned with long dangling braids. The students had begun to make fun of Lynn's parents as well. At that time her father was 57, and he had snow white hair. He had snow white hair as long as Lynn could remember. Those cruel elementary kids would ask Lynn if that was her grandfather. Lynn described those days as being emotionally abused by her peers. The other students would pull her hair and do all kinds of stuff to her. In the first week of school, she called her daddy because he was retired and home during the day. She was profusely crying and asking him to pick her up from school.

She gradually befriended a girl named Clara who had nine sisters and brothers. Clara became her angel and body guard. She would not let anyone mess with her. Lynn was an exceptional student who always managed to keep her grades up. By the time Lynn made it to middle school, her grades were still good but her behavior was unacceptable. A lot of her unacceptable behavior stemmed from her trying to fit in with other students. Lynn led a somewhat sheltered life. She was not allowed to attend parties, and she had to be in the house when the street lights came on. During this stage of her life, she had begun to get in a lot of trouble. The principal would call her mother, her mother would come to the school and beat her in the principal's office. She finally made it out of middle school and had entered into her high school years. Her high school years were even the more difficult, she was a very thin, flat chested teenager. Her friends had started to develop as young adolescents but not Lynn. Emotionally she was dealing with being skinny and flat chested because the boys were not paying her any attention as they were her other friends. She was still unable to attend parties, however, she was able to attend after school extra-curricular activities. All her friends had older siblings who introduced Lynn and her friends to drugs. At the age of fifteen Lynn had experienced illicit drugs such as marijuana for the first time. Lynn's father was physically challenged and would have frequent visits to the VA hospital. He would come back with a lot of pills which Lynn began stealing to take to school and distribute among her friends because she wanted to be accepted. She was able to get all her friends and herself high. As a result of getting high off her father's medications, Lynn passed out at school. With a 'BOOM' her body hit the floor. The school viewed her passing out as an accident and not as an adolescent student passing out in the hall as a result of drug use. The school officials did not know that she was abusing her father's medication. Lynn's behavior began to progress; she was still getting in trouble, and she had started cursing out her teachers. Regardless of her negative behavior she still managed to excel academically. She was active in the church where she served in positions such as usher, choir member, and was involved in various auxiliaries. Underneath all that Lynn still loved the boys. She would rebel by sneaking out the window to attend neighborhood parties and would not return home. As time advanced, she was in her senior year of high school, still exhibiting negative behaviors, and getting into trouble. The school officials told her that if she got suspended once again during her senior year, she would not graduate high school. All this time despite her troubled path, her grades kept her in school. Now the school officials were sick and tired of her; they were no longer concerned about her good grades because they doubted why they should try to save someone who does not want to save themselves. Needless to say, she did manage to progress some.

Just as things were getting better for Lynn, tragedy hit her home. On April 5, 1974, Lynn was awakened by a loud scream that penetrated the home from her mother's bedroom, telling her to call 911. After calling the emergency medical technicians, Lynn went into her parent's room to see what was happening and she saw her father on his knees beside the bed holding his chest in pain. Finally, the medics came to the home, took her father away and Lynn never saw her father alive again. She felt very alone since she and her mother never really had a relationship. She felt that her father was every breath that she took, she lived and breathed her father. He had always been the center of her universe. After her father died, she was no longer motivated to reach her goals. She managed to wander around and complete high school two months after her father passed away. During this time, she began excessively using marijuana. Lynn could not contribute her negative behavior and drug use to a learned behavior that she experienced in the home. She was never exposed to domestic violence, alcoholism, or drug addiction - not to say there were not any disagreements in the home, but they were not violent. Although her father was a military man and a deacon in the church, he was loving, caring, protective, and a provider when it came to his family. After high school, Lynn decided to move to Raleigh, North Carolina to attend King's College and she lived off campus near Mission

Valley in Raleigh. While in college she became promiscuous and very involved with a married man who was a coach at the college. After finding out he was married, she immediately left town and moved back home with her mother. After being home and having time to focus clearly on her life she decided to enroll in college at Fayetteville State University. Fayetteville, North Carolina is known as a military and party town. Being away from home gave her the freedom to make her own decisions and to do what she wanted to do. Lynn's party scene had increased. She was partying and drinking a lot. She was now at the club at least five days a week. During this time, she began dating a military officer from Fort Bragg, who was an excessive drinker too. It was the norm for soldiers to drink a lot but he did not approve the use of drugs. She began to drink with him even the more. Not only was she excessively drinking but she was very resourceful and she had found someone who sold marijuana, giving her the access to be able to smoke marijuana daily. Shortly after being at Fayetteville State University, she found out the officer that she had been hanging out and drinking with was married too. She decided that she was not going to be involved with someone else's man so she ended that relationship. Regardless of her negative behaviors, she was not into sneaking and hiding just to be with someone. Not long after she ended that relationship, she was out partying at this club and met the house DJ. It was an instant attraction. After dating for three to four months, he became the wardrobe manager for a popular 1970's soul-influenced funk group. This was when the downward spiral of cocaine use became a trend for her. This man paid for airplane tickets and limousines which transported her to New York to the studios where he worked. The supply of cocaine was plentiful. She was snorting cocaine in massive amounts. Being a college student no longer mattered to her. On Thursday nights and sometimes Friday mornings she would leave to meet him in New York. She began missing a lot of school due to not returning to school before her class started on Tuesdays. She noticed that her cocaine use was affecting her grades, but she managed to stay in school a little while longer. One day, she was hanging out and listening to the radio station where her man DJ'ed at and the station was congratulating him and his wife on their new baby. She was floored. That information really broke her heart. She thought he was different especially after the instant connection. She was tired of the abandonment and the lying. He was just like the guys she had dealt with in the past. Why would this man love on her like that, pay for airline tickets, limos, and other gifts and bring her to New York every week, only to find out that he and his wife were having a new baby. Men were plentiful for her; they came a dime a dozen. She was a young, attractive, sexy "red bone" with pretty hair. She appeared to have everything together. She was the IT girl back in the day. She was thinking, "One monkey won't stop her show." After ending her relationship with the famous wardrobe manager, she starting dating the golf pro at Fayetteville State University. She appeared to be in control of her addiction; no one knew she was using cocaine on a regular basis. Dating the golf pro was very different for her, in fact, he was too slow for her. She viewed him as being the poster child for doing everything right. She learned that maybe opposites do attract. Her life changed for the better for a short period while dating him. He was very involved in his education which made her take a look at where she was headed. She began to get more involved in taking control in terms of her education but after he graduated, she felt abandoned and alone again. She continued smoking marijuana and snorting cocaine.

The golf pro became a teacher at Livingston College and she visited him on some weekends. He had to attend a lot of functions so she became his arm candy. She knew she could not attend his functions high and she was bored after visiting him in his small town.

The one weekend that she did not travel to visit him, she was hanging out at The College Grill and she saw the guy she was purchasing her marijuana from. He noticed that she did not leave town that weekend. They began to talk. Not only was he her drug dealer, but he became her significant other. He too was a student at Fayetteville State University. He graduated and left just like the other men in her life from that area did. Lynn could not make that happen for herself. She did not know how to balance going to college and getting high at the same time, but all the men she met did what they needed to do to advance their career and move on. After her last boyfriend graduated, in the middle of her junior year, she decided to move off campus to move in with him. She always had her room on campus, but she was never there. He was still selling drugs and marijuana. In fact the guy he was purchasing his weight from went out of town and when he returned he had a mayonnaise jar filled with cocaine. At first they were just selling the powder cocaine, and they were making a large amount of money. She found herself being paranoid because of the massive amounts of drugs, and the shoe boxes full of money that was in the home. They started doing what they call free-basing, doing LSD, window pane, and other hallucinogens. She and her environment were out of control. They placed bars on all the windows, and a hole in the door to receive money and distribute drugs. It was like something you saw in the movies or in the slums of New York where massive drugs were being distributed. Her days had become consumed with getting high. She was not enjoying life; cocaine had consumed her life. Finally, they decided to get another apartment so that he would have a safe place to go outside of the dwelling where they were selling and manufacturing drugs. He found out the police were watching, and his spot had become hot. On the first and fifteenth of the month when the military got paid they made at least fifteen to twenty thousand dollars. She was harboring the drugs and money for her boyfriend. She would traffic a certain amount of drugs and money to the spot each day. One particular night they were invited to a house party, she and each of her associates were given an amount of cocaine to use at the party. After being high off of LSD, she was not ready to indulge in using her cocaine because she was already high. They starting gathering their works and cooking the cocaine until it became rock form, and she was mesmerized as to what they were doing. Her drug dealer boyfriend kept telling her that it was none of her business what they were doing and that she best not try it. That was the moment that she realized her drug dealer boyfriend was freebasing. One day the person they were getting their large supply from dropped by, and asked her to try something. Her boyfriend said no because both of them can't be smoking cocaine. She replied, "You can't tell me what to do." Lynn tried it and was instantly hooked; she fell in love with rock cocaine. Rock cocaine is 100% addictive for most people. She loved rock cocaine so much that she started stealing from the packages they were selling. She started cutting the packages so that it was not as potent and she and her boyfriend would have more to use together.

Things were going downward really fast; she went from being on top of the world to becoming homeless. She believes that cocaine affects women differently from men. She could not stay home or stay in, she went out in the street and sold her body to obtain more of the drug that she allowed to consume her life. Prostitution became the norm for her; she knew she could make the money she needed in order to obtain her drugs and support her habit, and she believed there were a whole lot of men in Fayetteville, North Carolina with a whole lot of money.

Due to chasing cocaine and trying to obtain the funds she needed to support her habit, she experienced her first sexual assault at the age of twenty-five. She was raped at knife point. She was so caught up in her addiction, knowing this man raped her, but she did not leave. She knew he had a lot of dope and money. She wanted that dope, and she stayed there with him after he raped her to get it. Her mindset and the disease of addiction told her to use him for what she could get out of him. He placed a knife to her throat, made her do and say things to him and he did horrible things to her that she could not control nor was she in agreement with. After this incident, she had dropped out of school, she still had her boyfriend, and she would still go out in the streets to cop her dope. Her mother knew something was wrong, but she could not put her finger on it. She knew her daughter was dating a drug dealer from Fayetteville, North Carolina, but she never said anything. She just wanted her baby girl to be happy. She did advise her not to marry him. Lynn did not listen; they thought they were so in love, and one weekend they drove to South Carolina and got married. Yes, they eloped. Afterward, they moved to New Jersey. She had obtained a job at Womack Army Hospital, and was later transferred to the Kennedy Center. She was twenty-seven years old and never worked, but she was making her way up the civilian rank in military services. Meanwhile, she was still getting high. It affected her work performance and attendance. She has the gift of gab so if she could talk to you, most of the time she could persuade you to change your mind no matter what the situation may have been. She was good at talking her way out of certain situations and consequences.

Lynn's sister-in-law was a prominent person in the Veteran Administration; she assisted Lynn in obtaining a job at the VA in Newark, New Jersey. She and her husband stayed with her sister-in-law until they secured their own place. Soon after they moved into their place they screwed up and made a bigger mess of their lives. Her husband who held a Bachelor's degree could not find employment; he was twenty- seven and had never held a job in his life. He then went into the military, and Lynn moved back to Hampton, Virginia with her mother until her husband got stationed in Fort Carson, Colorado. Her former drug dealer boyfriend who had become her husband had now become a military police officer. This was good and bad for Lynn. Military police officers would take people's drugs and let them off the hook, so now Lynn had access to drugs from all over the world. The supply had become plentiful again. She was living in Colorado which was a little over twenty-four hours from the Mexican border.

At that time, nothing was better for her until she found out she was two weeks pregnant. That was the day she stopped using cocaine for five months. Although she stopped using immediately after she found out she was pregnant, she could not suppress the urge any longer, and at five months she took a hit. The baby leaped so hard in her belly that it almost scared her to death. She did not use anymore during her pregnancy. She actually stopped using everything, but low and behold, the day that she delivered she was getting high in her hospital room. The baby was born at 1:11 pm and at 5:00 pm she was getting high. She did not want flowers, gifts, or candy, all she wanted was her dope. After the delivery of her baby, her husband was ordered to report to Istanbul, Turkey. Lynn decided that she and the baby would move back to Fayetteville, North Carolina, and she would return to work. Her plan was delayed due to her mother calling and asking if she could come home because she was not feeling well. She was still using, and she did not have any of the funds that her husband was sending her because her dope habit was consuming all of it. Her sick mother had to send her an airline ticket to get her home to assist her. She missed the first plane because she was busy getting high. Finally, she was able to arrive in Hampton, Virginia on a Saturday evening. The following Monday was Labor Day of 1985. On Tuesday, she transported her mother to the doctor, and the doctors informed both of them that she had brain cancer.

The news was devastating, and this led her to move home to take care of her terminally ill mother. The challenge of being a primary caregiver to her four-month-old child and her sick mother increased her desire to get high. She spiraled out of control and became a full-blown addict. Fortunately the military allowed her husband to return home and stationed him at Fort Monroe, Virginia in order to be with his wife during this challenging time. She then received news that her mother had two to four months to live.

Lynn's addiction was progressive; it never stopped expanding, but she was still there trying to take care of her mother. She was not able to leave her mother alone, but she had to get high.

The cravings were taking over, and she needed the drugs, therefore, she started getting high in her mother's house. Her mother was a few rooms down the hall from her. One particular night, her mother got up off her bed, she had been calling Lynn, who didn't hear her mother calling. She was in the utility closet getting high. Her mother must have smelled the stench of crackcocaine and ended up seeing her use drugs. This bothered her and she was saddened by it but nonetheless, she had to feed her addiction. She put that thought in the back of her mind and went forward each day chasing her addiction.

She loved Sundays, she couldn't wait until Sunday of each week. She knew the church folks would visit her mother, and they would always give her mother some money. Her mother placed the money in the Bible for safekeeping. Lynn started stealing her mother's money out of the bible. As time went on her mother got sicker. All she wanted was for Lynn's brother to take care of her; she knew Lynn needed saving, and she knew what was going on with her but she never said a mumbling word to her about it. Lynn felt that her mother never loved her like her father loved her and she always believed her mother loved her brother better than she loved her.

A week before her mother died, Lynn's baby came down with a really disgusting virus and had to be hospitalized. Her baby was in one city and she had to tend to her mother in an adjoining city. She was about to lose her mind; she was still getting high. Finally, the doctor came and reported that the baby was going to be well, and they could go home. Lynn was elated; she immediately called her mother. She could hear the sound of relief in her voice, it was if she was waiting for the baby to get well before she could go home to be with the Lord. One cold winter day, it was snowing really hard, and they had to go across the bridge and through the tunnel. Lynn was at the hospital tending to business that pertained to her baby. She felt in her spirit that something was wrong and she needed to go and see her mother. When they got to the hospital, she immediately knew as her brother stood up that their mother was gone. This was four months and seventeen days after the day the doctors gave her two-to-four months to live. Lynn was angry because her mother died while she was in the elevator coming to visit her. She was furious because she believed her mother wanted to be with her brother when she took her last breath. She was consumed with anger.

Now she was having regrets that her mother never had an opportunity to hold her baby girl; she saw her but was never able to hold her. Her mother was dead. She knew nothing about making funeral arrangements. She was able to get her mother buried but to this day she doesn't know how. The first call after she left her mother's bedside was to the dope dealer. She informed the dope dealer that her mom just died and he needed to bring her some dope "right now."

Two weeks later, her husband had to return to active duty in Istanbul, Turkey. He moved Lynn and the baby to Raleigh, North Carolina, because she could no longer stay in the family home where she grew up. There were so many good and bad memories there, and in her mind all she wanted to do was find another place to live. After getting settled in Raleigh, North Carolina, she was disbursing her mother's estate which was left to her, despite her drug using. She was making trips from Raleigh, North Carolina to visit her dope dealer in Hampton, Virginia, purchasing five to six thousand dollars' worth of dope at a time for a period of six months. In that period of six months, she had gone through one hundred thousand dollars. By the time her husband returned to the states from Istanbul, Turkey, she did not have any money. During this time, she would take her daughter to Virginia to her brother's house and leave her there for weeks at a time. They did not know if she was dead or alive. The home that she grew up in was a part of the estate she had received. She was an addict but sometimes the choices she made were not all bad. She decided to sign her mother's house over to her brother so that she would not smoke it up, and the dope man wouldn't get it. Even today her brother, his wife, and family still live in the family home in a prominent neighborhood in Hampton, Virginia. She is always welcomed there and will always have a place to call home.

A year after her mother died, Lynn still had her mother's checkbook and she began writing checks on her deceased mother's closed checking account. She was caught for forging checks and went to jail. Her brother and sister-in-law came to visit her for twenty minutes, left her twenty dollars, and left with her daughter. They did not get her out of jail. She made that bed and they made sure she would deal with lying in it. She was highly upset about that. She had given him a whole house; how dare he leave her? He could have put the house up for collateral to bond her out of jail. Her husband's commanding officers got her out of jail contingent upon her going to substance abuse treatment. She enrolled in inpatient treatment, was discharged on her birthday, which was the same day a guy in her treatment program got out. They went to celebrate her 30th birthday and this was the first time she started shooting cocaine. She went to a hotel with this guy and while she was smoking her dope, he was shooting his. She noticed his cocaine was lasting longer than hers. Therefore, she decided to try it. "It was the ultimate high." God was still so good to her. Even in the storm God was still working it out for her good. She was not able to shoot herself up because she has rolling veins and her veins were too small. She tried to shoot herself, and it didn't work. She later got connected with someone the people in the streets would call "The Doctor." He would shoot her up. One day he was shooting her up, and he used the cotton that he had been shooting his heroin with. She became sick as a dog. She was a cocaine addict, not a heroin addict.

She had started shooting so much it was hard to disguise. She was light skinned, and it was easy to see the track marks on her arm. After her husband saw the track marks on her arms, he began calling her a junkie. It pierced her heart and hurt her feelings so bad that she made a conscious decision never to indulge in shooting up again. By now her daughter had been in Virginia for a year with her family. As time moved on, she went back to Fayetteville, North Carolina. She had a few things going on, and she had become an entrepreneur of the streets. When people she knew would engage in breaking and entering, they would get checkbooks and bring them to her. She would write five to six thousand dollars' worth of checks on any given day. One night she had gotten greedy. She had been in Kroger once that day but she decided to go back. She had pre-written the check but had not signed it. While at the register an officer said, "Madam can we please have a conversation with you?" She went to jail and received twelve years in the North Carolina Correctional Center for Women in Raleigh, North Carolina. The checks kept coming in; she had written over twenty–six thousand dollars in checks. No one ever asked her if she had a drug problem, they would always say that she did not appear to be the kind of person that did the things she had been caught doing. God was still blessing her in spite of her negative behaviors. Instead of serving a 12-year sentence, they allowed her to complete 180 days in prison, five years of probation and a suspended sentence of six years. She completed her time and she was released.

On the 21st day after being released, she went to see her probation officer, cursed him out, told him that she was not doing five years of probation, and she wanted to be back in prison before it was time to order the Christmas boxes. Of course the probation officer looked at her with disbelief; he could not believe what his ears were hearing. By the end of that November, she was back in the North Carolina Department of Corrections for Women in Raleigh, North Carolina on a twelve-year sentence. She adjusted to the lifestyle of prison; it was business as usual for her. She had people who brought marijuana and cocaine into the prison for her, she was selling it to make money, loan sharking, still getting high, and she had gotten busted as well. She was an inmate and at the same time she was trying to run their prison system. When in Rome she learned to do as the Romans; she had a good relationship with some of the male guards. She had guards and sergeants who would break large bills for her because the inmates were only supposed to have thirty dollars at a time. At any given time, she might have a one hundred dollar bill. She was collecting money from the inmates who owed her money, some inmate's parents were putting money in her account because their child owed her money, and they were making payments for them. She was in prison but it was not her prison, she still had to follow the rules and face the consequences of not following the rules. At one time she was busted for having cocaine on the grounds. Once again, she was able to get out of it; the officers could not prove it was her cocaine.

There was one captain in the prison that believed in her when she didn't even see any good or potential in herself. Time advanced for Lynn and she finally was released from prison after doing almost five years under the old law and placed on intensive probation. She had gotten comfortable with living in prison and she was feeling defeated due to losing her daughter to her cousin who had gained custody. She was not allowed to speak with her over the phone, nor was her daughter allowed to write her. Surprisingly, she was allowed to travel home for Thanksgiving to see her daughter. This was not the norm for someone who was just released from prison to travel to another state. She went home and her immediate family took up a donation at the Thanksgiving table. She was able to get enough money for an attorney to try to regain custody of her daughter.

She and her husband did not get back together after she was released because she could not handle her husband getting another woman pregnant while she was in prison. She had already accepted the fact that he would probably be having sex with other women but the agreement was that he would not impregnate another woman. Therefore, she decided that they should live their lives separate.

After thinking back on her life, Lynn always knew she was an addict. She knew in prison, if she did not get herself together, she would not get her daughter. She knew that her only clean time had been while in prison. After doing almost five years in prison, she only had six months clean. No one ever offered her a drug program while in prison even though there were drug resources such as the DART program that was housed in prisons across the state of North Carolina. Lynn finally asked her case manager to allow her to enroll in the program or she would never be able to get her child back. The same year she was released, she asked her counselor Sally Marks daily to allow her into the program. She needed drug treatment. She had been active in her addiction since the age of 21. She had always known she was an addict. Her addiction caused her to engage in negative behaviors that included prostitution, stealing, stealing her child's gifts, stealing her mother's money, blowing her mother's estate, forgery, abandoning her child, quitting school, stealing from her employer, anything you can imagine that was negative Lynn has probably done it. She has done everything except kill someone. When she was active in her addiction, her family tried to deal with her. Her brother has always been very protective of her. At one time, her brother used to sell and she would steal his packages. She did not care who she stole from as long as she was able to feed her addiction. Back in the day, her brother was using marijuana, but he would never get high with her nor would he give her anything.

Her addiction was always a whirlwind. It lasted as long as it did because she always had men in her life who had money. People would always ask her why she was doing drugs in the streets. She spoke well, she was articulate, and she came from a middle-class family. She never told the girls she worked with on the streets that she was using drugs, she never got high in front of them, she would say that she had daughters in college, and she had to "make it do what it do" to get her daughters through college. Addiction has no barriers, name, race or gender. She had to get hers like the next addict, by any means necessary.

10 months after Lynn's release from jail, she finally got her daughter back. She met a man from the first NA meeting she

had attended and later married him. His name was Samuel Williams, and he was a Narcotic Anonymous (NA) guru and an employee of the Wake County Health Department and Southlight. He loved her and he helped her get re-established in the community. She has worked under some very prominent people and organizations in Raleigh, North Carolina including Passage Home (Jean Tedrow), Glory to Glory House of Refuge (Angela Ferrell Moss), Wake County Jail, and she was a member of the Wake County Continuum of Care.

After all that, things still weren't as she dreamed it would be. She thought things would be perfect. Little did she remember that life has its moments, and none of them are perfect. She instantly had to deal with life on life's terms. She had become fixated on the money, property, and prestige. She married this man because she needed someone who had stability, and he could help her get her daughter back. She loved him, but it was for the wrong reasons. One night after being clean for ten years she placed her kids in the bed, and she decided that she wanted to smoke some dope. She relapsed for one night. She came back and she stayed clean for three years. The next relapse started in her mind long before she made a decision to pick it up again. She started lying about her purchases, shopping, and other addictive behaviors. Her husband was always in the community helping others and providing support. That was his job. She was always home alone. She met this man that showed her a little attention and made her feel special. It was not questionable that her husband loved her, but he loved her with material things and she needed more practical things like affection and attention. That was the void that another man filled in her life, which led her to step outside her marriage, and she later moved out of her home. Although they tried to rekindle the marriage, it was not salvageable. That was the leading force that caused her to wake up the sleeping giant that was her addiction. At that point, her addiction progressed so quickly. She had fallen to an all-time low point in her life once again. This relapse caused her to stay in her act of addiction for an additional six years.

She was missing in action. Everyone was looking for her. Her pastor was looking for her. I remember driving all the streets that I knew had crack houses looking for her. She was my best friend; I loved and missed her. I would cruise the neighborhoods late at night hoping that I would run across her. At one time, she told me she saw me but she hid so that I was not able to see her. She had abandoned everyone. She abandoned her children, friends, husband, other family members, and she had abandoned me. She had pretty much abandoned everyone.

After she resurfaced again, her children had her committed to Holly Hill, a private mental hospital in Raleigh, North Carolina. They reported that she was suicidal, so she was admitted for thirty-one days. That still was not enough to change her addictive behavior. Shortly after being released from Holly Hill, she began living on the streets. She went from crack house to crack house. She became a full-time prostitute and thief. She went to jail here and there, but she had managed to escape prison for nineteen years. In 2006, she had received her first drug charge after all those years for maintaining a dwelling. Her drug dealer convinced her to get an apartment in her name. They promised she would have a regular supply of dope on a daily basis. The dope-dealer gave her a signing bonus and everything. In the beginning, everything appeared good. Later she found out that it was not enough - her addiction was calling for more than what the dope dealer was giving her. She would still have to boost and turn tricks to feed her habit. One morning at about 4:00 am someone knocked on the door and told Lynn that her daughter was outside and that she wanted her. She had been cruising the neighborhoods trying to locate her mother. She hugged her mother and said, "I know what you are doing, just promise you will stay in touch with me." Unusual things were happening to her during this relapse; things were going downhill. She was bitten by a pit bull; her house was raided while she was home, she was arrested for larceny, robbed in a drug house, and her friend was shot. Her life at the time was reckless and did not seem like it was going to get better. Her daughter was preparing to graduate from The University of North Carolina at Chapel Hill, her family had driven down to attend the ceremony from Hampton, Virginia, and she was not able to make the ceremony. She was in the hospital for eighteen days after being attacked by the pit bull. After the graduation ceremony, her family came to visit her. When she got out the bed, her family begin to cry after seeing how fragile, weak, and thin she had become. After leaving the hospital from the vicious dog bite, she still did not stop running the streets and getting high. She had gotten arrested again but she always knew God was her saving grace. She was glad she had gotten arrested. She needed that break and rest.

Due to being on probation for maintaining a dwelling, she went to prison for eight months. This was her second rodeo to prison. She was sentenced to Fountain Correctional Center for Women in Rocky Mount, North Carolina. While at Fountain, she went through another drug program called WRAP. After being released, she went back to the same crack house, and the vicious cycle started all over again for her. This time after being released from prison, she went out with a trick, and he cut her throat from ear to ear, busted her in her head, and she was walking down New Bern Avenue, in Raleigh, North Carolina bleeding like a slaughtered pig. Ironically enough, her ex-husband Samuel Williams saw her and transported her to Wake Medical Center. In her mind, she just wanted to get to the block to get high one more time before going to the hospital. She was released from the hospital with a drainage tube in her throat and immediately took a taxi to the block to get high. That still was not enough to stop her from using, but it changed how she did things in terms of turning tricks on the street. She had become paranoid. She started to pray and cry out to the Lord. She would say, "Lord, I no longer want to live like this anymore, please take it away." One brisk autumn day, while walking through Chavis Heights Park in Raleigh, North Carolina, she saw a group of people having a cook-out and she went over to ask for food. In her mind, she was going to get a plate for the dope man, with hopes that it would give her more leverage with him. Perhaps he would increase her dope supply. She went to the place where the people were gathering. One of the ladies in the group was Clara Downing Bain, the executive director at North Carolina Recovery Support Services (NCRSS). Clara hugged her, cried with her and asked her to come by her office on Monday if she wanted some help. She called and made an appointment, but she missed her first appointment. Nothing got better. Things had rapidly gotten out of control; she was homeless and ashamed. She made the second appointment. North Carolina Recovery Agency started picking her up every day for intensive outpatient groups. She would go to groups every day without food, after being up all night. They were literally picking her up from the crack house. She finally shared with Ms.

Clara that she wanted to change but she could not change without a place to stay. After Ms. Clara was able to secure Lynn a space in her sober living house, she has not found it necessary to pick up a drink or drug since her experience with the North Carolina Recovery Services. Lynn has been clean now for six years. The most rewarding accomplishment for her after being clean this time is she has been accepted back into Fayetteville State University, she is registered with the North Carolina Substance Abuse Board to test as a certified substance abuse counselor (CSAC), and her relationships with her children are totally different. Through it all she has become more open-minded and humble. For today, she realizes it is not about the money, property, and prestige. It's about staying clean one day at a time. She is not concerned about winning a popularity contest, she just wants to keep helping others and stay connected with the God of her understanding. Believing in God and working the steps to recovery in NA has been essential to the change in Lynn's life. Staying clean has become a lifestyle change for her. While dealing with her addiction, her biggest challenge was pride, and seeing people that she had provided services to in the community.

Getting back into the community without being self-critical and feeling guilt was also a challenge. Everyone knew her; she had been a community advocate for years, and she had worked as my assistant at Glory to Glory House of Refuge (Glory House) for many years. I was the founder and executive director of Glory House, and it was the only residential program for women living with HIV/AIDS, substance abuse, and mental health issues in Wake County, North Carolina for many years. Lynn was the second face of the organization in the absence of myself.

She could no longer run and hide from her disease. Over the years she learned that addiction seeks to kill, steal, and destroy. She embraces being a woman in long-term recovery today. This time around, she has been clean since October 15, 2009. She is thankful to her daughters, Chaunacie, Shasta, and granddaughter Samantha for continuing to believe in her and for loving her when she was not able to love herself, or when she didn't deserve their love. Lynn described her brother Ronnie as being the best brother a girl could ask for. She believes Ronnie's wife Richetta was ordained to be his wife. Through Lynn's addiction, her sister-in-law supported her husband's wishes for his sister and never allowed him to stop loving, caring for, and helping her. Her cousin Joy was able to care for her child so that she would not become a statistic of the foster care and welfare system. Lynn is forever grateful to her family and friends. She leaves one message for those who are struggling and are Dying to Live today. That message is, "You don't have to use drugs today, NO MATTER WHAT. The struggle is real but with assistance of agencies like North Carolina Recovery Support Services (NCRSS) and Oxford House in Raleigh, North Carolina, Recovery is REAL also!"

Fact: Drug addiction is a very complicated disease that many people in the United States struggle with. When an individual is trying to quit it takes more than good intentions or a strong will. Drugs alter the mind in ways that foster compulsive drug abuse, it is difficult to quit even if the individual has a mind-set to quit.

CHAPTER EIGHT

They Saw the Glory, but They Don't Know My Story

Beverly is a 53-year-old African American woman of God. She has two girls ages 19 and 30. The 19-year-old is currently in her sophomore year of college at Chowan University. The oldest daughter has a BA from North Carolina Central University. She was born in Goldsboro, North Carolina, and raised in the public housing project of Goldsboro. Beverly is the fifth of sixth children that were born to her single parent mother. Although she grew up in public housing in Goldsboro, she described life as being "…not hard, but good, as good as expected to be raised by a single parent with six children." Her father was murdered when she was two ½-years-old, which forced her mother to raise her and her siblings alone. Meanwhile, her siblings describe their life in another light where they lived a hard life. She does not recall life as being hard. She remembers not wanting for anything. In her mind, her mother took very good care of them, and they were good. She was never hungry, she was a cheerleader in high school, her uniform was paid for, and she was a straight "A" student, but her attitude needed modification. Her attitude was a U, but her grades were always an exceptional A. Her 1980 graduation class that year consisted of 460+ students, and she was number 101 in her senior graduating class. After high school, she did not have a clue of what she wanted to do with her life. However, the military recruiter she met in high school was always coming by to visit, and the frequency grabbed her. In her mind she was thinking she was not going into the military, she just wanted this recruiter to stop harassing her and leave her alone. That was her mindset at the moment. Later she made a decision to enroll in her area.

On July 27, 1981, three days before her 19th birthday she made a conscious decision to come to Raleigh, North Carolina so that the nagging recruiter could get credit for her recruitment. After listening to them and finding out she would be paid to be in the military she said, "OH shoot, if they are going to pay me for doing this, I am going into the military." She did not return to Goldsboro, North Carolina. She took the oath immediately, in fact, she took the oath right then and there on Saint Mary's Street in Raleigh, North Carolina. She immediately called her mother, and her mother's first response was, "You better not take my suitcase with you." She responded by saying, "Come and get it then." Her older sister who was currently living in Raleigh, North Carolina, and other siblings came to meet her at the bus Station on New Bern Avenue in Raleigh, North Carolina to see her off to the military. She was now officially an enlisted soldier. She did her basic training at Fort Jackson, and she graduated and became a full-fledged soldier. Beverly was a strong-willed and strong-minded person. Although the other new recruits were crying and breaking down, she stood her ground when it came to the military tactics the sergeants were using. In her mind she thought, "You don't know me, you don't know nothing about me or my mother," she was not going to break down and cry while they antagonized her. She was hard and she continued to stand strong as a soldier in the United States Army. In 1984, she was stationed in Germany and came back home to Goldsboro, North Carolina for visits; this is when she conceived her first child. After that, she returned to Germany but later returned to the States to deliver her baby girl. After having her daughter she had to relinquish temporary custody to her mother. As time advanced, she was stationed at Fort Bragg, North Carolina. That put her closer to her daughter. As time went on she got even closer to her child when she enrolled in the Army Reserve Unit in Raleigh, North Carolina on Garner Road. This was the good life; she was a professional independent woman living her life like it was golden. In 1996, she met a guy, they started dating, and she found out that he was a drug dealer. He was making that fast money. She did not need the money, but she liked the idea of it and the idea of having access to it. She knew he was selling drugs, but he would never allow her to use, he shielded her from the drugs and gave her the utmost respect when it came down to him selling his product, which was cocaine. He would never do anything around her. One particular day, she found his stash, and she was thinking, "Okay, so this is what it looks like." She had seen people use, but she had never experienced using. At that time she wanted to try it. She did not know what to do with it but she knew from seeing others that she had to transform it from powder form to rock form. She ended up destroying a lot of his product while she figured it out. After getting the cocaine to rock form, she tried it. In the beginning she did not like it, the feeling was strange, but she quickly became hooked. Her life had made a drastic change and before she knew what happened she was caught out there in her addiction for four years. She realized she was a crack cocaine addict when she had to send her child back to live with her mom in Goldsboro, North Carolina due to being evicted from her housing in Raleigh, North Carolina. When she went to Goldsboro to take her daughter she was trying to be incognito. At that time, she thought she was better than the next addict because she had not advanced to the other negative behaviors that addicted women were doing, like selling their bodies for drugs. She had her own money and did not have to do that.

Beverly described her addiction as being different because she was not in the streets. Once she thought everyone was inside she would go out in the streets to get her hit. Crack cocaine had become her best friend for four years. She did not look like the average crack head, she had somewhere to go, she had a roof over her head, and she made sure her hair was on point. She took a bath every day. In fact, she thought she was cute. While in her active addiction her second child was conceived, and she was smoking crack cocaine every day. She did not want her baby to be born addicted to crack cocaine so she decided to smoke once a week. She thought that she had it under control. She thought she knew how frequently to smoke crack cocaine so that it would not affect her unborn child.

While being active in her addiction, her siblings did not turn their backs on her. For a long time, she was their go to person. Her mother always knew she was getting high, but she never judged her nor did she talk down to her. In fact her family would give her money and say now don't get high with that money, and she would boldly say to them, now what do you all think I am going to do with this money? I am surely not going to pay any bills with it. Beverly knew not to be in her mother's presence high, and to this day her mother has never seen her high. She knew that her mother was constantly praying for her. In November of 1998, she received the message that her mother was sick with cancer. No matter where she was or what she had done she was always there on time to sit with her mother while her sister went to work. She had lost her job as a paralegal assistant with a local attorney in Goldsboro, North Carolina due to her addiction consuming her.

In January of 1999, she experienced another hardship that took her down a spiraling slope. Her mother had passed away. She was able to be there to see her mother's last living breath taken. After the death of her mother, she was thinking her life could be much better than living a life of an addict. She used for a few more months, but little did she know that God was turning things around, and he had a plan for her life. In June of 2000, she returned to Raleigh, North Carolina to Wake County Alcoholism Treatment Center. The staff told her that she needed to come back in 24 hours, and she immediately responded, "I will be sitting right here when my 24 hours are up." She was trying to explain to the staff that if she left she would go out to get high. The staff informed her that she could not sit there and she did not fit the criteria for treatment. She asked, "What is the criteria for treatment?" They said she had to be a threat to self. Beverly exited the treatment center, and proceeded to walk into oncoming traffic on New Bern Avenue (a high traffic area), hoping that a car would hit her. She was not hit by a car, in fact, the drivers took precaution so that they would not hit her. She then reported back to Wake County Al-coholism Treatment Center and informed staff that she had Suicidal Ideations and she walked into traffic on New Bern Avenue with hopes of getting hit by a car. After returning to the treatment center, they accepted her into their inpatient treatment program. When she had a week left in inpatient treatment, she had no clue what she would do after treatment. One day, I came to the treatment center to interview women for the Glory to Glory House of Refuge. I accepted Beverly into my program and she says Glory House saved her and kept her safe.

Beverly's children were never exposed to her addiction. Her older daughter was shielded from all of it by her grandmother, aunties, and uncle. Her younger daughter was being raised by her father. In June of 2000, she began to cry out to God, "Lord, please deliver me and take the taste of crack cocaine away from me." God immediately saved her. We were having Bible study at Glory to Glory House of Refuge, and they also took the girls to church. That is when her church life and real relationship with God started. God helped her. She knew about NA and other self-help programs, but God was the source of her deliverance.

Her most rewarding accomplishment since she has been clean is seeing her oldest daughter graduate from college, seeing her younger daughter enter into her sophomore year of college, growing spiritually and growing in her relationship with her daughters, being reintegrated back into society with dignity and hope as well as being a homeowner and working numerous years in state government. She has learned coping skills to deal with the changes she was facing and she has also learned not to be impulsive. Today, she has a choice; she is not going to be treated and spoken to in any kind of negative way. She has learned to put herself in time-out to be able to walk away from situations and later return and address the situation in a cordial and peaceful way. She feels like she had to take this path in life to help others to come out. People see the glory in her life, but they don't know her story. She is a servant at heart, and she embraces those who struggle with addiction when they come into the ministry where she serves. She also believes that church folks can be the most critical people. If someone doesn't look or smell a certain way, they don't want to be bothered with that person. In her church she makes sure she embraces those in the struggle and she lets them know that they are not alone. If needed they call on her for a listening ear and a shoulder to lean on. Of the many responsibilities she has, she still finds time to give back by volunteering with the North Carolina State Prison System. Today, Beverly has been clean fourteen years and she is honest enough to admit that there have been times that she wanted and thought about going out to get high. To Beverly, recovery is work and is sometimes a constant battle between the flesh and the spirit. Her main deterrents that keep her from getting high is breaking the heart of her children and the fact that she has made a choice not to go back because she is chosen by God to be a royal priesthood, and she does not have to live that life anymore. The one message that she would like to leave to encourage those struggling with addiction is that you can come out from under that stronghold. If you want help, it is there for the getting, because a changed mind can lead to changed ways.

Fact: In 2006, there were 6 million Americans aged 12 and older who abused cocaine in some form. 1.5 million people had abused crack cocaine at least once in the year prior to being surveyed.

CHAPTER NINE

Mental Illness and ME

Mental Illness in North Carolina is not unusual. In 2010, of the 9.2 million people living in North Carolina, approximately 335,000 adults live with a serious mental illness and 99,000 children also live with severe mental illness. The stigma that is associated with mental illness is as extensive as the stigma that is attached to HIV/AIDS. Having a stigma about HIV/AIDS and mental illness is unfortunately common. There are also many stereotypes towards these individuals that cause discrimination. It is assumed that people with mental illness are impulsive, unstable, and engage in violence. These individuals are judged by others and are constantly judging themselves. Because of the stigma attached to being mentally ill, sometimes individuals will not engage in treatment, are not open about discussing their mental status, the lack of understanding of their illness from friends and family members is frustrating to them, they have limited opportunities such as school, work, and housing, they are victims of bullying, harassment and crime, they have inadequate health insurance, and they believe they that can never manage their disease well enough to be normal. I would like to introduce Jessica. I have known Jessica all her life; she is my little cousin. Jessica was born in Raleigh, North Carolina to a single parent. She has three siblings whom she adores. Jessica was raised by her mother who later thought it was best that she go to live with her grandmother, grandfather, aunt, and uncle who were all living in the same home. They ended up co-parenting her until she became old enough to move out on her own. Jessica's mother thought it would be best if she was raised by them because she was going through her own struggles at that time. While Jessica was growing up next door to the home where I grew up, and was going through her adolescent years, I had already married and moved away from home. Currently, Jessica is living in Fuquay Varina, North Carolina as a single 29 year old woman living with bipolar and emotional distress. Although others are ashamed to discuss mental illness due to the stigma that is still attached to having mental illness today, Jessica is bold about telling her story. Jessica tells her story with hope that it will empower others and she tells it with power and authority. She says her teenage years were complicated and difficult due to not having her mother and father with her. She had other people that she could talk to or go to but it did not have the same effect as having her mother and father there with her. She was not able to do average things that normal teenagers were able to do like going to amusement parks, or going to high school games and activities. She was never allowed an opportunity to try out for sports or do other things like go to the beach. She was very good in volleyball and basketball, but she did not have the support from her parents to join a team. When she was in the Gospel choir, they liked that because gospel singing was something they liked and embraced. It was not like they had a lot to do, she was the only child for eight years. After eight years, her mother had a son.

She felt from the day her brother was born until now, her mother has paid her little attention and has not given her any affection. She was hurt by being sent to live with her grandparents and auntie. After that transition, she felt unwanted, and later she felt safe because of her grandfather; he was the main role model in her life. She thought she had done something wrong which caused her mother to send her away. She felt like she was being punished by being sent to live with her grandparents who did not do anything for fun. "It was almost like being sent to reform school," she said. When she first attended high school at Garner Senior High, it was wonderful, then suddenly tragedy happened in her home. Her grandfather passed when she was a freshman in her second quarter of high school, which put a strain on her and caused things to change in her life. Her grandfather was her role model and the only male figure in her life that she trusted and depended on. Despite the struggle that year, she was able to pass her ninth grade year and attended the new high school in Apex, North Carolina called Middle Creek High School. While at Middle Creek High School, things changed for her, she was not doing well in school at all. She started experiencing negative behaviors such as staying out of school and being unfocused. She felt like nothing was the same for her anymore after having lost the only role model in her life. Everyone else was doing their own thing and she felt like she was alone. Things were constantly going downhill for her. During her sophomore year at Middle Creek High School she was expelled for assault. At the time her education was still an important factor for her, and she later enrolled in a re-direct type of educational program at Mary E. Phillips High School in Raleigh, North Carolina. This school assisted individuals who had struggles and experienced behavior issues, giving them an opportunity to complete their high school education outside of the traditional school schedule. She had become a junior at Mary E. Phillips High, which was exciting to her because she was able to be placed in her correct grade. Although it seemed like things were looking up for her something was still wrong because she made a decision to drop-out of high school during that year. She was not motivated and felt as if she had nothing to live for. School no longer had her attention. She was not able to do things on her own, there were many barriers there that included lack of motivation, and no support from her mother and father. Shortly after she had noticed that something was different about her, she wasn't even interested in doing things that usually interest her. She felt like she did not have a purpose in life, and she felt hopeless. After dropping out of high school, she decided to enroll in Job Corps Career Training program in 2004. Even though she was not in school, education was still on her mind; she had hopes of being a doctor or lawyer just as other adolescents. She decided that Job Corps would be good for her because of the structure. Little did she know that Job Corps would not work for her either, she had lost her attention span once again. Staying focused was a major issue for her. She had tried many things, she just could not seem to put her finger on why she was not able to stay focused. In 2005, she experienced an emotional breakdown. She attempted suicide after a 12-year relationship ended. He was the apple of her eye, the one person she could depend on who always had her back. He gave her things she wanted and needed. When he could not provide things for her he showed her how to grind and go get it for herself. He was her best friend. When the relationship ended, she felt like everything she had was gone. During that breakdown she was diagnosed with bipolar and emotional distress. She also suffers with anxiety and other phobias, has crying and sleeping spells, and becomes violent, emotional and confrontational. Life had become really bad for her. She developed a really bad attitude. She never abused illegal drugs, but she did have to attend Alcohol Anonymous (AA) for excessive alcohol use. Jessica started exhibiting reckless behavior due to not being able to cope, and her non-compliance with taking medications escalated the situation along with the excessive drinking. She was not consistently taking her medication; it was difficult for her to do because she had overdosed on pills twice. She also had a third overdose of alcohol poisoning, which led her healthcare providers to recommend outpatient substance abuse treatment, and she complied. Her suicidal attempts stemmed from family issues; she felt she was the black sheep of the family, and she was never given encouragement or support by her family. She felt like she never had the family she needed or deserved. Her overdose was never for attention, she really wanted to check out. She would have been alright with dying from those attempts. Even after the attempts, her family still did not seem to care nor did they come to see her. Sometimes they would accept her phone calls and sometimes they would not answer. For them, it was life as usual. Coming from a broken home may have been one of the factors that caused a lot of her illness, frustration, and negative behavior.

As she increased in age those negative behaviors seemed to manifest even more. She started stripping and became an entertainer for Big Beautiful Women (BBW) entertainment. This company traveled and provided strippers for different occasions. That was one of the ways she acted out. She enjoyed it because everyone knew her name and her photo shoots were gorgeous. She was getting attention, she was traveling and getting paid and that felt good to her. She didn't think she would have had access to those things outside of BBW entertainment. This was a part of her acting out mentally. She realized she was getting older and she wanted to grasp hold of her reckless behavior. She loved money but she knew she had to let it go, she could no longer live that lifestyle after stabilizing her mental illness.

For her stripping was an addiction and it created the same behaviors that addicts experience while using drugs. She did not realize what she was doing or had done until she completely came down from the high of stripping and entertaining. Later her colleagues would tell her some of the things she was doing, and she was in disbelief that she behaved in such a negative way, beneath her values and the morals that her grandparents had taught her. She was able to keep her stripping on the low for a long time. After her family found out about it, some did not have a problem with it and thought she was bold to engage in such behaviors. Stripping boosted her self-esteem and it gave her confidence. She had the mind-set that she was a BBW (big beautiful woman) and sexy too.

Other behaviors she engaged in when she was hurting was getting piercings, tattoos, and shaving either side of her head. This was a part of her self-harming behavior. When she pierced her body, it took away her emotional pain. She has 15 piercings and 22 tattoos. She is constantly in this cycle that needs to be broken. She believes she's had an undiagnosed mental illness since the age of ten and has been in this vicious cycle for nineteen years. She's been in treatment for many years but was not on psychotropic medications. Her siblings are also currently going through the same issues as she did. One of her sisters and her brother are diagnosed with mental illness.

People who are struggling with a mental illness have ups and downs. They need somebody to talk to, someone to manage their medications in order to make sure they are taking them, proper sleep, and a structured environment. When individuals with mental illness feel like they have no one, this tends to make communication difficult because they feel like everyone is against them and they are alone. It took Jessica a long time to figure out that the struggles she was dealing with were warning signs and complications from her undiagnosed mental illness. After her family was made aware of her situation, some family members tried to get along with her and offered assistance, others thought it was funny and they made fun of her situation because she had to take Seroquel, Cymbalta, and Trazadone. This made Jessica upset but later she came to an understanding that it was not about them, it was about her. She recognized she was sick and needed treatment. Today, she is still engaged in treatment with Wake County Human Services. The comments Jessica's family made are no longer important to her, she is the most important person in her own life. Jessica felt that coming from a middle class family, this was not supposed to happen to her. She had goals and ambition. Her mother found it difficult to understand her behavior as well, but she was supportive in terms of getting her to treatment. Mental illness has no boundaries; both sides of Jessica's family struggle with mental illness. Jessica thinks that her mental illness is hereditary. The maternal side of her family has a high incidence of depression and anxiety. The paternal side of her family struggled more with addiction than mental illness.

Completing her education is still a goal for Jessica. She is in the process of enrolling in Wake Technical Community College to complete her high school education. Since learning of her mental illness, she has not allowed it to keep her from becoming successful. She has obtained her certification in medication administration, NCI Interventions, and nursing assistant. The biggest challenge of having a mental illness for her is being able to manage her daily tasks, medication compliance, and following through with things. She copes with her challenges by engaging in treatment, talking to others, and applying the coping skills she has learned in treatment.

Mental illness is complex and not the laughing matter that many people make it. Jessica's message is that people with mental illness sometimes need an ear or a shoulder, just listen to them. It is not always appropriate to try to offer advice. Just Listen. These types of people are always seeking someone they can confidentially entrust their information to without judgement. They are seeking that person who can be there for them as a strong support. Just be quick to listen and slow to speak when dealing with a person who lives with a mental health issue. Over the years, Jessica has engaged in services from Triumph Behavioral Health in Raleigh, North Carolina and Wake County Human Services. Triumph provided exceptional services to her until their funds were cut. This left her with limited mental healthcare, and poor coordination of care. Through it all she learned to manage her illness and is living a productive life with dignity and hope.

Fact: Mental and substance abuse disorders are the leading cause of disability worldwide. About 23% of all years lost contributed to disability is caused by mental illness and substance abuse disorders.

CHAPTER TEN

AIDS, Substance Abuse, and Mental Health Issues: What Else Can a Girl Ask For?

Carla is the sister of two brothers. She was not aware that her father had another child outside of marriage until her adolescent years. Carla came from a very dysfunctional family where abuse and domestic violence was prevalent. Carla's father was abusive to her mother, while her mother was the glue that kept the family together by working two to three jobs. Carla's dad was not a provider, he did whatever he wanted to do while her mother worked her fingers to the bone in order to provide for the family. He was not even a responsible caregiver for the children while her mother worked. The onset of childhood trauma started when her biological brother who was ten years older than she was sexually molested her while her mother was at work.

Eventually, Carla's mother got tired of raising her family alone with no support from her husband. She finally made a decision to divorce him. Carla, her mother, and her older brother ended up moving forward with their lives. Her mother continued to work numerous jobs, but she was able to receive assistance from her younger brother and a neighbor. The support aided in helping to keep the family together and life became a little easier for her mother after people stepped in to assist her with raising her children. Low and behold, at the age of fifteen, Carla became pregnant. Her mother thought she was able to support Carla and her child so she could complete school but she quickly found out she was not able to do so. Carla had to quit school to assist with raising her child during her sophomore year. Later Carla began to feel like her mother never had time for her because she stayed busy all the time, and she was always working. Carla was always seeking the love and acceptance of her mom, hoping to gain her approval. She remembered getting off the school bus one day as a little girl and running up to her mother saying, "Mom look what I did, look what I made," and her mom would always say, "Um-hmm." She never received the uplifting and praise that she wanted and expected to receive from her mother. As her life went on she was always looking for love and approval. In school she was buying her friends; she felt like if she gave people stuff, they would become her friend. Buying friends and seeking acceptance consumed her life for a very long time.

Carla never returned to school. She obtained her GED while in prison in 2007. She was very intelligent and was always seeking to enroll in college classes and taking trade oriented courses during her time of incarceration. After looking back at her life, she remembered her second-grade teacher meeting with her mother to suggest that she could benefit from counseling but her mother went off on the teacher after she made that suggestion. The teacher was aware that something psychological was wrong with her. Her mother knew at that time she was dealing with some psychological issues, but instead of giving her the treatment she needed she decided to continue living in denial concerning Carla's mental health issues.

Carla believed that her life always has been an embarrassment to her mother. She knew her mother loved her, but she didn't express her love like Carla wanted her to. Her mother loved her the best that she knew how and expressed it the only way she knew. After making her last bid in prison in 2010, she saw that her mother was making some changes in how she engaged with her and how she viewed life. She later learned that her mother's changes were due to her accepting Jesus Christ as Lord and Savior in her life.

Carla and her brother were never brought up in a church. Her mother used to send her and her brother to church with the neighbor on holidays. Now that her mother accepted Christ, she and Carla finally had a mother and daughter relationship and get along better today. Carla's mother is still in denial though concerning some of the things that have happened to Carla during childhood.

As an adult, Carla tried to tell her mother about the sexual abuse from her brother. Her mother told her to "shut up," and said she didn't ever want to hear that come out of her mouth again. There were a lot of pink elephants in the room in Carla's house. She was forbidden from discussing her childhood and other trauma that took place in her life. She did not know about bipolar, depression, anxiety, schizophrenia, and other mental illnesses. Carla started embracing her mental illness later in life after she started dealing with her substance abuse, but as a little girl, she was morbidly obese, and she started finding comfort in food and looking for acceptance from people.

She then started to use drugs; it was strange to her, but she liked it. She liked the way it made her feel, but she did not understand what the drugs were doing to her. She attempted suicide on her 21st birthday. She had never had a birthday party in her entire life. When she turned 21, she got together with some friends and threw a birthday party for herself. She had engaged others who were doing drugs and this was her first time trying it. She found herself smoking cigarettes, smoking weed, drinking, and the whole nine yards. This was October 1989. Between December and February of 1990, she had spent $30, 000 wastefully in drugs. This was also the first time she engaged in substance abuse treatment. During that time she was dually diagnosed and found out she was bipolar. She still did not understand exactly what was going on with her. She struggled with her mental illness and substance use for many years. She did not take the time to take a close look at her issues; she did not take the time to learn about those issues.

It took Carla a long time to become concerned about her substance abuse and mental illness issues. In fact, it took her longer to embrace the mental illness because she never took the medications. She self-medicated by using drugs or by engaging in crazy relationships. Her history was when she felt like she was going crazy or couldn't take it anymore she would give it up for a while and for some reason she would always go back to self-medicating. One day she asked herself if she was going to wake up to see what the problem was or was she going to keep going through the problem?

In 2014, she had an epiphany. She was tired of going through the motions of addiction, and unmanaged mental illness. By this time, she had been through 25 years of addiction, mental institutions, jail, prison, a halfway house, and special needs programs. She had been looking for any and everything to fix Carla but she was stuck in a revolving cycle of drugs and relationships. Three years ago, she gained a strong relationship with the God of her understanding. He began to break some chains in her life. After a period of time God began to deliver her from the attachment of being in a relationship with men, he helped her with managing her mental health condition, but the chain of her dope addiction had not been broken at that point. Although the dope chain was not broken, Carla never gave up. She gave out a few times, but she never gave up. She says she "could feel the strength of God." When she was caught in the web of life and felt she was trapped, she knew that all she could do was to call on the name of Jesus. When she did not know who to call on she would say, Jesus, Jesus, Jesus, and He never failed to show up; He would always calm her storm.

Her greatest challenge of dealing with her mental illness was the fact that she was noncompliant with taking her medications. It was difficult for her to stay on course with her mental health regimens. She would always fall into the mode of self-medicating with drugs. The depression would allow her to fall so deep into a fog that she could not come out; she was feeling helpless and hopeless. She has now learned how to deal with managing her mental illness. Her whole mind-set has changed. Romans 12:2 states, "Be not conformed to this world: but be ye transformed by the renewing of your mind, that ye may prove what is that good, and acceptable, and perfect, will of God." This is how she is coping with mental illness today. Today she has built an alliance of people in her life she can call on and ask for help. She had gotten fed up with herself, and came to the realization that no one can help her until she realizes that she needs help and she has to acknowledge that she needs help before she can receive it.

Carla has tried to take her life so many times. When she found out she was HIV positive, to her it was the end of her life. She began to plead with God by asking, "Why me? Why did I have to be the one infected with HIV/AIDS?" The spirit of the Lord spoke to her and said, "Why not you?" Carla has been living with the knowledge of having HIV for 24 years. She learned of her status while in prison. Her greatest challenge of dealing with HIV has been self. If she gets beyond herself, she can begin to lead a self-directed life with dignity and hope. No one in her life has a problem with her status; they still love her. So what is the issue? She has a strong support system; she has resources, and she is attending clinical trials and obtaining medical services at UNC hospital systems. UNC Hospital is one of the best hospital systems in the country. Not only that, she found the love of her life, her fiancé. She is currently in a mixed status relationship (her partner does not have HIV) with plans to marry soon. With all those positive things going on she still tends to worry about dying when one of her opportunistic infections tends to flare up. HIV/AIDS is real. It is still here. She sees it as a constant reminder but when she is in a funk she can call on one of her supportive friends who is also HIV positive. She gains motivation from that friend and settles her spirit by saying if her friend can do it, then she knows that God will also give her the strength to endure her pain, disappointment, and storms.

Today her name is no longer "HIV", her name is Carla Louise Bridges. It's no longer crack head, mental patient, bitch, slut, or whore, her name is Carla. She no longer cares about who people say that she is, she knows who God said that she is, and nothing else matters to her. Her thoughts are if God loves her, why she can't she love herself? At one time she was blinded by the devices of the devil but God has given her access to the light and the chain of dope is now broken from her life. All her life she believed lies and believed what people said she would be but now the truth has made her free. She no longer has to lie, when truth prevails. Carla has learned how important it is to focus on who you are and not who people say that you are. HIV/AIDS is a chronic disease but it can be managed. Carla is no longer dying inside but she has chosen to live. Make a choice to live and know your status.

Myth- Mental Illness is cause by a personal weakness.

Fact: *No one is at fault for having a mental illness, it is caused by environmental and biological factors, not a result of personal weakness.*

Nami.org-National Alliance on Mental Illness.

Very Present Help

Whether these women are living with HIV/AIDS, substance abuse, or a mental health issue, they are still women who need to be respected, loved, and cherished. They are our mothers, sisters, aunties, cousins, grandmothers, and daughters. Before anything else, they were a little girl who grew up to become a woman. Life can be a constant battle for women, so to add in other variables such as HIV/AIDS, substance abuse, and mental health issues, can be devastating. These women have experienced rejection from family members, friends, church groups, and human services providers. Their rejection has caused some of them to slowly open up about their conditions, but has caused other women to become silent in the struggle of living with HIV/AIDS, substance abuse, or having mental health issues. These issues often have stigma attached that result in rejection and isolation within their own families and among their peers.

Each woman highlighted in this book dealt with different struggles but one thing they all had in common was that their behaviors put them at risk of contracting HIV/AIDS. The women who did not have HIV/AIDS shared negative behaviors such as prostitution and abusing substances and they were not mentally competent enough to understand that what they were doing could cause them to become infected. Each of them spoke about God's saving grace over their lives. They did not wake up one day and say they were going to live reckless lives. The paths they took were predestined and in the end God had an obstacle course planned out for them. The women's positive lifestyle changes increased their life span, they have reintegrated back in to the community and workforce and they have tremendously improved their quality of life. All of the women acknowledge Jesus as their Lord and Savior and no longer shall they die but they shall live and declare the works of the Lord (Psalm 118:17). These women believe that some need church support and others need AA or NA in addition to the church support. All the women who were residents of Glory to Glory House of Refuge's supportive housing program benefited from both the services we were offering at the facility, their local churches, and the Serenity programs that were hosted at our facilities.

As the founder and executive director, I was introduced to Ruth, a community substance advocate and her late husband Preston Wooten, founders of Serenity in 1998. Ruth had been a community advocate for many years in terms of empowering those with substance abuse and other issues. Their program was so impressive that our organization started hosting Serenity meetings at our facilities six years after their program started. Ruth spoke a word into the atmosphere one night and God heard her supplication. Ruth's husband was an alcoholic and she had been attending Al-Anon's self-help group. Al-Anon's goal is to offer assistance to friends and family of problem drinkers with understanding and support. Ruth was sitting at home one day after having attended a few Al-Anon groups, and she was thinking "wow," it would be nice if she had a Christian-based support group to assist her with dealing with her current situation. Her husband had been out on a binge that night. As she was sitting there watching TBN, God showed up with a message about support groups for believers who were struggling with addiction. Ruth immediately located a Christian-based support group in Raleigh, North Carolina. She attended the group three times a week for several months. That was the

birthing of Serenity, the group that she and her late husband
Preston Wooten co-chaired together. Serenity is a self-help
group in Raleigh, North Carolina that assists Christian believers who are struggling with addiction. The group's foundation
is the word of God. Serenity was created and started July 4,
1990. Immediately after starting the group, Preston's binges
stopped and he became clean from that day forward. Since the
inception of Serenity, this Christian-based self-help group has
and still is changing the lives of many men and women in Raleigh, North Carolina. Serenity groups follow the same steps as
Narcotic Anonymous (NA) and Alcohol Anonymous (AA) but
what separates this group is that it stand on the foundation of,
"Therefore if any man is in Christ, he is a new creature; the old
things are passed away; behold all things have become new" (2
Corinthians 5:17). Serenity and programs such as Serenity that
have a Christian foundation to assist the body of believers is
needed. No one is exempt from the possibility of struggling
with disease of addiction. While providing services to the
women and men of Raleigh, North Carolina, Ruth was able to
understand more about the disease as she focused on her past
struggles of abusing prescription medications to hide the things
she did not like about herself. She was enlightened about the
progression of this powerful disease called addiction. Most of
the women who were in the program were doing the same
things. They turned to drugs to cover up things that they did not
like about themselves. They lived their lives behind masks for
many years. Serenity allowed them to unveil and as they re-
moved pieces of their masks, truth was revealed and God was
delivering them at the same time. Later they were able to gain
confidence. They no longer had to live behind the mask and
they could now live and not die. They were "Dying to Live"

but very few people saw that and were willing to assist them. Preston and Ruth saw beyond the veil and offered them assistance through Serenity.

Serenity has changed the lives of many in Raleigh, North Carolina. This program has proven to be very effective, and Ruth stated that some of those who participated in the program have become pastors, ministers, and drug counselors. The resident women of Glory to Glory House of Refuge participated in Serenity programs for over nine years. Some of these women are now homeowners, working state and government jobs, have become professionals, leaders in their church and community, and most of them are still living clean and sober today. Even after the passing of the late Preston Wooten, God still uses Ruth to provide Serenity services to individuals and groups who request the services. Ruth and I believe that churches should embrace women and others who are struggling with HIV/AIDS, substance abuse, and mental health issues. We also believe that people with these struggles should acknowledge the SIN, focus on the "I" in the middle of sin, and learn that the cure for it all is Jesus Christ.

AIDS Resources

Snap Shot of HIV/AIDS from 1981 to 2015

1981

- In 1981 the Centers for Disease Control and Prevention (CDC) in the United States reported the first cases of rare pneumonia in young gay men. This was the beginning of the HIV/AIDS epidemic in the United States (The Henry J. Kaiser Family Foundation, 2015).

1982

- In 1982 the Center for Disease Control and Prevention (CDC) was able to establish a name for this disease. The name Acquired Immune Deficiency Syndrome (AIDS) was launched to the world (The Henry J. Kaiser Family Foundation, 2015).

1983

- In 1983 the AIDs candlelight ceremony was held for the first time. During this time, the Public Health Service of the United States also presented issues for preventing transmission of the AIDS infection through sexual contact and blood transfusions (The Henry J. Kaiser Family Foundation, 2015).

1984

- In 1984 the Department of Health and Human Services (HHS) in the United States announced that Dr. Robert Gallo of the National Cancer Institute found out that a retrovirus causes AIDS. Dr. Gallo and Dr. Luc Montagnier of the Pasteur Institute held a joint press conference to announce their findings. The retrovirus was identified as HTLV-III, they later re-named it to Human Immunodeficiency Virus (HIV) (The Henry J. Kaiser Family Foundation, 2015).

1985

- In 1985 the first International AIDS Conference was held in Atlanta. The conference was hosted by the Unites States Health and Human Services and the World Health Organization (The Henry J. Kaiser Family Foundation, 2015).

1986

- In 1986 current President Reagan first mentioned the word AIDS in public, and the first panel of the AIDS Memorial Quilt was created (The Henry J. Kaiser Family Foundation, 2015).

1987

- In 1987 the first antiretroviral (ARV) drug — zidovudine or AZT (a nucleoside analog) was approved by U.S. FDA, and the United States Congress approved $30 million dollars for emergency funding to states for AZT to treat HIV/AIDS (The Henry J. Kaiser Family Foundation, 2015).

1988

- In 1988 the first national World AIDS Day declared by World Health Organization (WHO) on December 1st (The Henry J. Kaiser Family Foundation, 2015).

1989

- In 1989 there was a foreign traveler who was not allowed in the United States due to having AIDS. It was reported on ABC World News April 6, 1989. During this time the United States Congress created a National Commission on AIDS (The Henry J. Kaiser Family Foundation, 2015).

1990

- In 1990 the Americans with Disabilities Act (ADA) was enacted by United States Congress; which prohibited discrimination against individuals with disabilities, including people living with HIV/AIDS. (The Henry J. Kaiser Family Foundation, 2015).

1991

- In 1991 NBA basketball star Earvin "Magic" Johnson announced he is HIV-positive and retired from basketball (The Henry J. Kaiser Family Foundation, 2015).

1992

- In 1992 the United States Federal Drug Administration (FDA) licensed the first rapid HIV test, which provides test results in as little as ten minutes. (The Henry J. Kaiser Family Foundation, 2015).

1993

- In 1993 Unites States President Clinton established the White House Office of National AIDS Policy (ONAP) (The Henry J. Kaiser Family Foundation, 2015).

1994

- In 1994 AIDS became the leading cause of death for all Americans ages 25 to 44 and remained so through 1995. (The Henry J. Kaiser Family Foundation, 2015).

1995

- In 1995 the first White House Conference on HIV/AIDS was held. (The Henry J. Kaiser Family Foundation, 2015).

1996

- In 1996 the number of new AIDS cases diagnosed in the United States declined for the first time in the history of the HIV/AIDS epidemic. (The Henry J. Kaiser Family Foundation, 2015).

1997

- In 1997 AIDS-related deaths in U.S. decreased more than 40 percent compared to prior years, largely due to HAART (Highly Active Antiretorial Therapy) (The Henry J. Kaiser Family Foundation, 2015).

1998

- In 1998 the first large-scale human trials (Phase III) for an HIV vaccine began. (The Henry J. Kaiser Family Foundation, 2015).

1999

- In 1999 the United States Congressional Hispanic Caucus, with the Congressional Hispanic Caucus Institute, convenes Congressional hearing on impact of HIV/AIDS on

Latino community (The Henry J. Kaiser Foundation, 2015).

2000

- In 2000 the President Clinton created the first ever Presidential Envoy for AIDS Cooperation. (The Henry J. Kaiser Family Foundation, 2015).

2001

- June 5th, 2001 marked 20 years since first AIDS case was reported. (The Henry J. Kaiser Family Foundation, 2015).

2002

- In 2002, HIV was the leading cause of death worldwide among those aged 15-59. (The Henry J. Kaiser Family Foundation, 2015).

2003

- In 2003, President Bush announced the President's Emergency Plan for AIDS Relief (PEPFAR), this was a five-year, $15 billion initiative to address HIV/AIDS, TB, and malaria in hard hit countries. (The Henry J. Kaiser Family Foundation, 2015).

2004

- In 2004 the United States Federal Drug Administration (FDA) approved OraQuick Rapid HIV-1 Antibody Test for use with oral fluid; oral fluid rapid test granted CLIA waiver (The Henry J. Kaiser Foundation, 2015).

2005

- In 2005 the first National Asian and Pacific Islander HIV/AIDS Awareness Day in United States was created (The Henry J. Kaiser Family Foundation, 2015).

2006

- In 2006, June 5th marked a quarter century since the first AIDS cases were reported. (The Henry J. Kaiser Family Foundation, 2015).

2007

- In 2007 President Bush called on Congress to reauthorize PEPFAR at $30 billion over a 5 year period (The Henry J. Kaiser Foundation, 2015).

2008

- In 2008 the Center for Disease Control (CDC) released new HIV incidence estimates for the United States, showing that the U.S. epidemic is worse than previously thought. (The Henry J. Kaiser Family Foundation, 2015).

2009

- In 2009 President Obama called for the first-ever National HIV/AIDS Strategy for U.S. (The Henry J. Kaiser Family Foundation, 2015).

2010

- In 2010 President Obama's Administration released its first comprehensive National HIV/AIDS Strategy for U.S. (The Henry J. Kaiser Family Foundation, 2015).

2011

- On June 5, 2011 it marked 30 years since first AIDS case reported (The Henry J. Kaiser Family Foundation, 2015).

2012

- In 2012, the United States Federal Drug Administrations (FDA) approved OraQuick, the first rapid test that uses oral fluid that can be bought over-the-counter. (The Henry J. Kaiser Family Foundation, 2015).

2013

- In 2013 the UNAIDS (United Nation AIDS) reports that since 2005, deaths related to AIDS have declined by almost 30% (The Henry J. Kaiser Family Foundation, 2015).

2014

- In 2014 major coverage reforms under the Unites States Affordable Care Act went into effect, this impacted health coverage for many people with HIV in the United States. Also a child who was thought to be HIV-free after medication tested positive for HIV, which was a disappointing setback for those fighting for the cure (The Henry J. Kaiser Family Foundation, 2015).

2015

- In 2015 the findings from "Strategic Timing of AntiRetroviral Treatment" (START) study release showed that starting antiretroviral treatment early improves health outcomes for people with HIV (The Henry J. Kaiser Family Foundation, 2015).

North Carolina HIV/AIDS: Did You Know?

An estimated 36,300 people were living with HIV infection in North Carolina (including 6,500 individuals who may not be aware of their HIV infection), as of December 31, 2013.

In 2013, Mecklenburg (31.0 per 100,000 population), Edgecombe (31.0 per 100,000 population), Cumberland (26.0 per 100,000 population), Durham (25.7 per 100,000 population), and Guildford (23.5 per 100,000 population) counties had the highest rates of newly diagnosed HIV infections among the 100 counties in North Carolina.

HIV-related deaths ranked as the 23rd most common leading cause of death in North Carolina in 2013.

In 2012, North Carolina was ranked 15th in the nation, including the District of Columbia and US dependent areas, for the estimated number of persons living with AIDS.

Texas HIV/AIDS Statistics

In 2014, the number of women living with HIV in Dallas, Texas at the end of the year was 1,090.

In 2014, the number of women living with AIDS in Dallas, Texas at the end of the year was 1,074.

In 2014, the number of women living with HIV in the state of Texas at the end of the year was 8,417.

In 2014, the number of women living with AIDS in the state of Texas at the end of the year was 8,933.

North Carolina Mental Health Statistics

In North Carolina's approximately 9.2 million residents, close to 335,000 adults live with serious mental illness and about 99,000 children live with serious mental health conditions.

In 2006, 1,106 North Carolinians died by suicide. Suicide is almost always the result of untreated or under-treated mental illness.

Nationally, we lose one life to suicide every 15.8 minutes. Suicide is the eleventh-leading cause of death overall and is the third-leading cause of death among youth and young adults aged 15-24.

North Carolina's public mental health system provides services to only 34 percent of adults who live with serious mental illnesses in the state.

North Carolina spent just $126 per capita on mental health agency services in 2006, or $1,105.4 million. This was just 3.1 percent of total state spending that year.

In 2006, 74 percent of North Carolina state mental health agency spending was on community mental health services; 25 percent was spent on state hospital care. Nationally, an average of 70 percent is spent on community mental health services and 28 percent on state hospital care.

In 2006, 1,029 children were incarcerated in North Carolina's juvenile justice system. Nationally, approximately 70 percent of youth in juvenile justice systems experience mental health disorders, with 20 percent experiencing a severe mental health condition.

In 2008, approximately 8,200 adults with mental illnesses were incarcerated in prisons in North Carolina. Additionally, an estimated 31 percent of female and 14 percent of male inmates nationally live with serious mental illness.

The average rent for a studio apartment in North Carolina is 84 percent of the average Supplemental Security Income (SSI) payment, making housing unaffordable for adults living with serious mental illness who rely on SSI.

North Carolina Substance Abuse Statistics

Drug rehabilitation and substance abuse treatment admissions for the state of North Carolina statistics are broken down into these categories of primary drug abuse or addiction, age group, & cultural background (2015).

NORTH CAROLINA		Total	Alcohol only	Alcohol with secondary drug	Cocaine (smoked)	Cocaine (other route)	Marijuana	Heroin	Meth
Total	No.	32,999	10,754	6,095	4,669	1,040	6,547	839	185
	%	100.0	32.6	18.5	14.1	3.2	19.8	2.5	0.6
SEX									
Male	%	70.0	77.1	72.7	60.1	60.9	71.8	61.4	54.1
Female	%	29.9	22.9	27.3	39.8	39.0	28.2	38.4	45.9
Unknown	%	0.0	0.0	0.0	0.0	0.1	0.0	0.2	0.0
Total	%	100.0	100.0	100.0	100.0	100.0	100.0	100.0	100.0
AGE AT ADMISSION		0.0	0.0	0.0	0.0	0.0	0.0	0.0	0.0
0-11 years	%								
12-17 years	%	8.5	2.1	3.9	1.0	2.3	30.3	0.7	7.0
18-20 years	%	6.2	2.7	5.3	2.5	4.9	15.4	5.1	11.9
21-25 years	%	12.2	9.0	12.0	8.0	13.2	19.5	13.7	20.0
26-30 years	%	13.0	11.3	13.7	16.0	15.9	12.0	16.2	19.5
31-35 years	%	14.9	13.9	16.3	22.6	20.7	8.8	14.8	13.0
36-40 years	%	16.4	17.1	20.5	24.1	18.6	6.6	15.1	14.1

41-45 years	%	13.0	16.4	15.0	15.4	12.5	4.1	14.2	8.6
46-50 years	%	7.7	11.4	7.9	6.7	6.9	1.8	13.5	1.6
51-55 years	%	3.7	7.0	2.8	2.3	2.0	0.7	4.5	2.7
56-60 years	%	2.0	4.5	1.1	0.7	0.7	0.3	1.4	0.0
61-65 years	%	0.8	2.1	0.4	0.1	0.3	0.0	0.4	0.5
66 years and over	%	0.8	1.9	0.2	0.0	0.0	0.0	0.1	0.0
Unknown	%	0.7	0.6	0.6	0.6	2.1	0.7	0.2	1.1
Total	%	100.0	100.0	100.0	100.0	100.0	100.0	100.0	100.0
RACE White	%	59.2	63.0	60.5	39.9	55.1	56.2	56.9	91.9
Black or African-American	%	34.8	27.5	35.2	55.9	40.6	38.4	39.0	4.3
American Indian or Alaska Native	%	2.0	1.6	1.9	2.6	2.1	3.1	1.1	1.6
Asian or Native Hawaiian or Other Pacific Islander	%	0.2	0.2	0.1	0.1	0.2	0.4	0.1	0.0
Other	%	3.2	6.7	1.8	0.8	1.7	1.5	2.5	2.2
Unknown	%	0.6	1.0	0.5	0.6	0.3	0.4	0.5	0.0
Total	%	100.0	100.0	100.0	100.0	100.0	100.0	100.0	100.0
ETHNICITY Hispanic or Latino	%	2.9	6.3	1.4	0.6	1.7	1.4	2.1	1.6
Not Hispanic or Latino	%	93.0	89.2	95.6	95.2	94.2	95.2	93.1	95.1
Unknown	%	4.1	4.5	3.0	4.2	4.0	3.4	4.8	3.2
Total	%	100.0	100.0	100.0	100.0	100.0	100.0	100.0	100.0

End Notes

AIDS Chicago. (2016). Condom Effectiveness: The Facts about HIV and STD Prevention. Retrieved from http://www.aidschicago.org/resources/legacy/condoms/ltoyw_fact.pdf

AIDS Institute. (2015). Where did HIV come from? Retrieved from http://www.theaidsinstitute.org/education/aids-101/where-did-hiv-come-0

AIDS.gov. (2015). What are HIV and AIDS? Retrieved from https://www.aids.gov/hiv-aids-basics/hiv-aids-101/what-is-hiv-aids/

AIDSMap. (2016). Zidovudine Retrovir. Retrieved from http://www.aidsmap.com/resources/treatmentsdirectory/drugs/AZT-zidovudine-iRetroviri/page/1730919/

Avert. (2015). HIV and AIDS among African American. Retrieved from http://www.avert.org/hiv-aids-among-african-americans.htm

Bacon, O. (2005). HIV/AIDS for Veterans and the Public. Retrieved from http://www.hiv.va.gov/patient/faqs/risk-of-sex-with-positive-person.asp

Cocaine Addiction Facts. (2015). National Referral Center for Cocaine Addiction. Retrieved from http://www.cocainedrugaddiction.com/cocaine-information/cocaine-addiction-facts

Marks, N. F., Jun, H., & Song, J. (2007). Death of Parents and Adult and Physical Well-Being: A Prospective U. S. National Study. Journal of Family Issues, 28(12), 1611-1638.

National Institute on Drug Abuse. (2012). Understanding Drug Abuse and Addiction. Retrieved from http://www.drugabuse.gov/publications/drugfacts/understanding-drug-abuse-addiction

North Carolina State Statistics. (2010). Retrieved from http://naminc.org/nn/misc/NCstats.pdf

North Carolina Substance Abuse Statistics. (2015). Retrieved from http://nationalsubstanceabuseindex.org/north-carolina/stats.php

Smith, M. (2011). Study: H.C. Among 10 States with Highest HIV Infection, Death Rates. Retrieved from http://www.indyweek.com/news/archives/2011/12/08/2721357-study-nc-among-10-states-with-highest-hiv-infection-death-rates

Ten Facts about Mental Illness. (2015). Retrieved from http://www.who.int/features/factfiles/mental_health/mental_health_facts/en/index1.html

The Henry J. Kaiser Family Foundation. (2015). Global HIV/AIDS timeline. Retrieved from http://kff.org/global-health-policy/timeline/global-hivaids-timeline

WebMd. (2015). the Top 10 myths and misconceptions about HIV and AIDS. Retrieved from http://www.webmd.com/hiv-aids/top-10-myths-mis-conceptions-about-hiv-aids#2

Weinberg, R. (2004). 34: Len Bias Dies of Cocaine Overdose. Retrieved from http://espn.go.com/espn/espn25/story?page=mo-ments/34

About the Author

I have worked in the human services field serving homeless individuals living with HIV/AIDS, substance abuse, and mental health issues since the early 1980s. I have a genuine love for people and a desire to empower people to make positive behaviors changes as I have. I am the mother of two, Travis O. Ferrell II, and Mya Moss. I currently hold a Master's in Psychology and a Ph.D. in Health Psychology from Walden University. I will practice my discipline as a Health Psychologist in Fort Worth, Bridgeport, Decatur, and Denton Texas. Over the years, I have achieved a lot of awards for my dedication as a service practitioner. Those awards include Strengthening the Black Family Award, John Hope Franklin Humanitarian Award, JC Penny Golden Rule Award, North Carolina Hero Jefferson Award, North Carolina Interagency Council for Coordinating Homeless Programs Award, North Carolina Community Development Corporation Practitioner Award and the Jacki London Ministries (JLM) Practitioner of the Year Award. My greatest professional accomplishment was when I founded and opened a non-profit organization called Glory to Glory House of Refuge (Glory House). Glory House was a transitional housing program that served single homeless women living with HIV/AIDS, substance abuse, and mental health issues. The organization was opened from June 1998 to October 2007 until I resigned to obtain my undergraduate degree. After my resignation, the board of directors could no longer operate the program, therefore, the doors of the organization were closed. My second greatest professional accomplishment was graduating from Walden University with a doctorate degree in health psychology. Thirdly, is the publishing and launching of this book, *Dying to Live.*

I am currently residing in the Dallas, Texas area. I love being married to Wayne D. Moss, Jr., and traveling to spend time with my family and friends in North Carolina. Not only that, I enjoy providing services to individuals. I can be reached at www.AnjelaMoss.com.

Made in the USA
Middletown, DE
13 November 2022

14837189R00086